D0406541

Understanding Crohn Disease a

Understanding Health and Sickness Series
Miriam Bloom, Ph.D.
General Editor

Understanding Crohn Disease and Ulcerative Colitis

**Jon Zonderman
and
Ronald Vender, M.D.**

University Press of Mississippi
Jackson

www.upress.state.ms.us

Copyright ©2000 by Jon Zonderman
All rights reserved
Manufactured in the United States of America
08   07   06   05   04   03   02   01   4   3   2
∞

Illustrations by Regan Causey Tuder

Library of Congress Cataloging-in-Publication Data

Zonderman, Jon.
   Understanding Crohn disease and ulcerative colitis / Jon Zonderman
and Ronald Vender.
      p. cm.—(Understanding health and sickness series)
   Includes bibliographical references and index.
   ISBN 1-57806-202-0 (cloth : alk. paper)—ISBN 1-57806-203-9
(pbk. : alk. paper)
   1. Inflammatory bowel diseases—Popular works.   I. Vender,
Ronald.   II. Title.   III. Series.
   RC862.I53 Z66 2000
   616.3'44—dc21   99-052483

British Library Cataloging-in-Publication Data available

Contents

Preface and Acknowledgments

When I left full-time newspaper work in 1981 for a career as a freelance writer, a former journalism school professor gave me some good advice. "Write about what you know," he said. In my earliest discussions with the editor of this series, Miriam Bloom, I suggested a number of possible books, but told her I would most like to do a book on inflammatory bowel disease. She agreed.

I later told Dr. Bloom that I had been diagnosed with Crohn disease in 1988, and that the physician I had chosen to assist me as a collaborating expert author was the gastroenterologist who has provided my care since then.

My recollection of broaching the subject of working together on this book with Dr. Ronald Vender is vivid. It was December 1997, in an examination room in his new office. Since the previous February I had been fighting the worst flare-up of Crohn disease I had ever experienced. We had tried to beat back the attack with high doses of my standard mesalamine drugs—Asacol and sulfasalazine, three different antibiotics, steroids, and immunoregulators.

During the previous ten months I had been hospitalized twice for medication-induced pancreatitis; had endured weeks of liquid diet and canned nutritional supplements; had undergone barium X-ray studies, a CAT scan, and an ultrasound; had struggled with the pain, fatigue, and precipitous weight loss of the disease and then with the bloating, weight gain, and mood disorders of steroid treatment. My family had suffered with me.

Low-dose steroids had not held the disease at bay; at this meeting we were bumping the dose up again, and Dr. Vender advised me to schedule surgery to relieve the obstruction in my ileum that was the cause of the immediate crisis. I asked him to pull research materials for me as quickly as possible, so that I could work on the project while recuperating from my surgery.

Today, I am feeling much better. This project has been, to some degree, an exercise in healing as well as one in better understanding. I hope it provides the same benefit for others who suffer from Crohn disease or ulcerative colitis.

I am indebted primarily to four people for their assistance on this effort.

Thanks to Miriam Bloom for allowing me to write about what I know and for all her kind guidance and gentle criticism over the past fifteen months, from our earliest discussions at the American Medical Writers Association convention in Boston, through the structuring of a tight and coherent outline, and on to a finished manuscript.

Deep thanks to Dr. Ronald Vender, both for his collaboration on this project and for his many kindnesses during the eleven years he has practiced the "art of treatment" of my Crohn disease.

Thanks are also due to Dr. Melissa Perkal, a good friend, the surgeon who performed my surgery, and a terrific teacher who in many informal discussions helped me understand the ramifications of the full range of surgical treatments for IBD.

Finally, thanks to my wife and personal physician, Dr. Laurel Shader, who not only read the final manuscript with both her medical eye and the critical eye of the literature major she was in college, but who has lived with and suffered from my condition nearly as much as I.

J. Z.

When Jon Zonderman first approached me about assisting him on this project, I was delighted. As an author and a physician's spouse, Jon has always had interesting and perceptive observations to make about his illness and its treatment, and we shared the philosophy that "patients should be patients as little as possible." We believe in a collaborative approach to medical care that encourages the patient to live as full and independent a life as possible. While this book is largely the result of Jon's efforts, I would like to thank him for the contributions I was allowed to make.

A number of colleagues, past and present, deserve my thanks. First I would like to thank my former teachers at Yale. In particular, my mentor, Dr. Howard Spiro, first encouraged me to be interested in inflammatory bowel disease. I am indebted to my colleagues at the Hospital of St. Raphael in New Haven, Connecticut. This marvelous community teaching hospital is a model for sophisticated, compassionate health care. I would especially like to thank Dr. Peter Herbert (chief of medicine), Dr. Charles Riordan (vice president for medical affairs), and Sister Ann Virginia (former CEO of the Hospital of St. Raphael). I would like to thank my many colleagues in the New Haven and Milford medical communities who have honored me with their referrals. Many of them have been role models of caring and compassion, and I value their friendship.

My partners and staff deserve special thanks. They have allowed me the freedom and independence to pursue my interests and passions. Ms. Ann Gamble, my secretary, has skillfully organized and directed my professional life for over ten years. I am blessed to work with an outstanding group of physicians including Dr. Andrew Bedford, Dr. Dean Chang, Dr. Matthew Cohen, and Dr. Renu Umashanker. I particularly need to single out and thank my longstanding partners, Dr. Mark Taylor and Dr. Frank Troncale. Dr. Taylor, the editor of two textbooks on gastroenterology himself, combines academic excellence and remarkable patient care better than anyone I know. My friend and close colleague, Dr. Troncale, and I have now practiced medicine together for almost eighteen years. Dr. Troncale is the former chief of gastroenterology at the Hospital of St. Raphael, and he continues to be a role model for me as a caring, dedicated, and effective clinician.

More than anyone, my family deserves my thanks. My parents, Earl Vender and the late Muriel Vender, always provided me with love, support, and encouragement. My son, James, a student at Boston College, has been a great companion and great son. I appreciate his patience, support, and love. Amy, my wife of twenty-five years, cannot be adequately thanked in words. She has been my best friend, best companion, and greatest supporter. Thank you.

Finally, I would like to thank all of my patients. It has been my great privilege and pleasure to serve as their physician. I thank them for their continued trust and support.

R. V.

Introduction

Crohn disease and ulcerative colitis are inflammatory bowel diseases (IBDs) of undetermined cause. The diseases strike rich and poor, men and women, whites, blacks, and Asians. It is most frequently diagnosed in individuals between fifteen and thirty years of age. The Crohn's & Colitis Foundation of America (CCFA), the national organization that coordinates much research on inflammatory bowel disease, extrapolates from epidemiological studies of small populations that between 750,000 and 1 million Americans suffer from IBD.

A number of other types of colitis (inflammation of the colon, or large intestine) exist; among them are colitis brought on by certain medications or infections and ischemic colitis, caused by a lack of blood flow to the colon.

While the causes of Crohn disease and ulcerative colitis are not known, our understanding of the immune system and the mechanisms of inflammation within the bowel has led to improved treatment of both conditions since the 1970s. Some researchers look for a genetic or molecular key that will unlock the mystery of Crohn disease and ulcerative colitis; others seek medications that relieve symptoms and have fewer side effects than those currently in use. On the surgical front, new techniques for connecting a healthy small intestine to the rectum mean that fewer people who undergo total colectomy (removal of the colon) must live with an ostomy (an opening in the side of the abdomen for removal of waste).

Ulcerative colitis can be "cured" through a total colectomy, but Crohn disease has no cure. Crohn disease is a lifelong, recurring disease, even after surgery to correct an obstruction, an abscess, or a fistula (an irregular pathway from the intestine to another portion of intestine, to another organ, or to the outside via the abdominal wall). People who suffer from IBD, and especially those with Crohn disease, are likely to experience the emotional and psychological anguish associated with a chronic illness that can flare up at any time, changing one's short-term and even long-term plans.

Inflammatory bowel disease affects men and women in almost equal numbers. Northern European countries have a higher prevalence than southern European countries; in the north the rate approaches that of America and Canada. Jews of Ashkenazic (European) descent—about 90 percent of the North American Jewish population—have the highest incidence.

Inflammatory bowel disease in North America is more prevalent in the white community than among blacks or Asians. Black Americans have a higher incidence than Africans, and Asian Americans have a higher incidence than Asians. The rate among the Japanese is rising, bringing that population closer to the levels found in America and northern Europe than in the rest of Asia.

This book is written for all those interested in ulcerative colitis and/or Crohn disease—for those who have the disease, their families and friends, and their coworkers, as well as for teachers and camp counselors who interact with children and teens who have either disease. For those stricken as children or in their teens, the diseases can be especially traumatic, both physically and emotionally.

The diseases tend to strike when we are at our most vulnerable, between the ages of fifteen and thirty, when we are moving toward independence and beginning to form new family relationships, and between fifty and sixty-five, when we are looking forward to our peak working years and then to the pleasures of starting to wind down.

We begin this book as an individual or a family member might begin an experience with ulcerative colitis or Crohn disease—with a trip to the doctor and a search for the cause of the diarrhea, sometimes with blood in the stool, or of the severe abdominal pain, which might be chronic or intermittent, sharp or crampy, and is especially bad during the night or immediately after meals.

Next we move to an overview of how the healthy digestive

system functions and then to an explanation of how the digestive system malfunctions in an individual with ulcerative colitis or Crohn disease.

We go on to the topic of living with ulcerative colitis or Crohn disease, including a discussion of how to "know thyself" and understand the early symptoms that signal an impending flare-up, as well as what some of the short- and long-term extraintestinal (outside the intestine) symptoms are. We look at the special situations of inflammatory bowel disease in children and in the elderly, and at issues surrounding inflammatory bowel disease and reproductive function, both in women and men. The discussion of symptoms and effects of the disease leads to one of treatments, both medical and surgical. A host of new medications has become available since the beginning of the 1990s, and more are at all stages of the drug development pipeline. Surgical techniques also continue to improve.

Psychological and emotional issues deserve special attention. For many years in the middle of this century, inflammatory bowel disease was believed to be psychosomatic (a physical manifestation of a psychological problem). While certain chronic organic conditions can be psychosomatic, medical evidence has shown that this is not the case with inflammatory bowel disease. However, there is a strong link between exacerbation of the underlying disease and increased stress.

Increasingly since the 1980s, gastroenterologists who research the conditions and treat those who suffer from them have come to understand and appreciate the delicate mind/body relationship and the ways in which emotions and psychological frame of mind can influence the course of a flare-up, how well treatment works, and the general quality of life for an IBD sufferer. Chronic illness, sometimes with repeated hospitalizations and frequent surgeries, can be devastating not only to the individual who suffers but to the entire family. We firmly believe that individuals who suffer from either Crohn disease or ulcerative colitis can do much to improve their emotional and psychological capabilities for facing the disease, and thus can actively improve quality of life.

The last chapter contains a brief discussion of the research being done on possible causes and treatments of ulcerative colitis and Crohn disease.

This book draws heavily on a number of resources. For a basic text we used the fourth edition of *Inflammatory Bowel Disease,* edited by Joseph B. Kirsner, M.D., Ph.D., and Roy G. Shorter, M.D. (Williams & Wilkins, 1995). The second edition of *Inflammatory Bowel Disease: A Guide for Patients and Their Families,* edited by Stanley H. Stein, M.D., and Richard P. Rood, M.D. (Lippincott-Raven, 1999) is an official publication of the Crohn's & Colitis Foundation of America (CCFA). Lippincott Williams & Wilkins also publishes the official journal of the CCFA, the quarterly *Inflammatory Bowel Diseases*, which we consulted heavily. In addition, the CCFA's quarterly magazine, *Foundation Focus,* is a helpful resource; each issue contains an article about current research, as well as practical "how-to-live" information on such issues as obtaining health, life, and disability insurance. *Immunology: A Short Course* (second edition) by Eli Benjamin, M.D., and Sidney Leskowitz, M.D. (Wiley-Liss, 1991) was also helpful.

The National Foundation for Ileitis and Colitis (NFIC), the organization that preceded the CCFA, published three books in the 1980s that are still helpful today. They are *The Crohn's Disease and Ulcerative Colitis Fact Book,* edited by Peter Banks, M.D., Daniel Present, M.D., and Penny Steiner, M.P.H. (Charles Scribner's Sons, 1983); *People . . . Not Patients: A Source Book for Living with Inflammatory Bowel Disease,* edited by Penny Steiner, M.P.H., Peter Banks, M.D., and Daniel Present, M.D. (self-published by NFIC, 1985); and *Treating IBD: A Patient's Guide to the Medical and Surgical Management of Inflammatory Bowel Disease,* edited by Lawrence Brandt, M.D., and Penny Steiner-Grossman, M.P.H. (Raven Press, 1989).

Other books that may be useful are *Crohn's Disease & Ulcerative Colitis,* by Fred Saibil, M.D. (Firefly Books, 1997) and *The Angry Gut,* by W. Grant Thompson, M.D. (Plenum Press, 1993). See appendix B for a more complete reading list.

Understanding Crohn Disease and Ulcerative Colitis

1. Diagnosing Inflammatory Bowel Disease

Most people don't see a doctor about stomach pain or a little diarrhea. They expect that each year they will be hit with the "stomach bug" a couple of times. Also, literally thousands of cases of mild "food poisoning" occur annually that are not documented. Short-term gastrointestinal illness seems to be the lot of modern humans. But if the diarrhea and pain persist for more than a few days, most people go to the doctor.

When a doctor examines a person with gastrointestinal illness, his or her first thought is not of inflammatory bowel disease. Rather, until tests show that the condition is serious, the doctor's initial assumption is that the individual is suffering from a viral or bacterial illness or possibly from a parasitic infection. Many of these illnesses resolve themselves in a few days, or respond to simple treatments. It is only after a number of such bouts, or when the pain is severe, or the illness is accompanied by sudden and severe weight loss, or blood appears in the stool, that the doctor looks for something more serious.

The Difficulty of Diagnosis

The diagnosis of inflammatory bowel disease may be made quickly or may take a relatively long period of time, depending on the symptoms people have when they first visit a doctor because of distress. These signs (what the doctor finds) and symptoms (what the patient experiences) vary, depending on whether the inflammatory bowel disease is Crohn disease or ulcerative colitis and on where in the digestive system the disease is located.

Onset of symptoms of either disease can be sudden and strong or slow and subtle. Many symptoms are similar to those of other gastrointestinal illnesses, which can complicate diagnosis. In some instances an individual with either disease may become quite ill within a few days or even several hours. But more often the symptoms progress over a period of weeks or months.

In order to make a diagnosis of Crohn disease or ulcerative colitis, a doctor needs to take a careful medical history, perform a thorough physical examination, and possibly order a number of laboratory tests and diagnostic procedures.

Although the outward symptoms of Crohn disease and ulcerative colitis are often the same, the ways in which the diseases manifest themselves both within the gastrointestinal tract and throughout the body are very different, as we will see in chapter 3. As knowledge grows about how the two diseases behave differently at a cellular level, treatments are increasingly differentiated (this will be discussed in detail in chapter 5).

Inflammatory bowel disease is diagnosed most commonly in two age ranges: from adolescence to young adulthood (ages fifteen to thirty) and in middle age (fifty to sixty-five). Individuals in either age group may be reluctant to get medical attention for what they may consider to be intermittent bouts with diarrhea, abdominal pain, and cramps, but they should not be. Prompt diagnosis and treatment of inflammatory bowel disease is important. These are chronic, lifelong conditions and demand medical vigilance so that the best possible quality of life can be maintained. In addition, those in their fifties are entering the age at which colo-rectal cancer becomes more prevalent; it is important that individuals be evaluated by a physician who can distinguish colitis from cancer.

The History

An adult with undiagnosed inflammatory bowel disease may show up in a doctor's office with any number of symptoms and complaints. But three classic symptoms that a doctor looks for in assessing whether an individual suffers from inflammatory bowel disease are persistent or recurrent diarrhea (with or without rectal bleeding), pain, and fever.

Diarrhea

Diarrhea, sometimes accompanied by rectal bleeding, can be caused by a number of illnesses, including bacterial and viral ones, as well as by parasites. Diarrhea occurs because of a disruption of fluid transport through the intestines caused by a disturbance to the gut epithelium. Diarrhea can be organic (caused by disease) or functional (caused by abnormal contractions of the smooth muscle that makes up the intestines). Before they make a diagnosis of inflammatory bowel disease based on a single bout of diarrhea, even a persistent one, it's important for doctors to rule out these more transient causes.

The most common cause of diarrhea is acute viral gastroenteritis, the second most common disease in the United States after upper respiratory viruses. Most of us are familiar with the symptoms—nausea, vomiting, diarrhea, low-grade fever, abdominal cramps, and muscle pains. To many people, these viral infections fall under the catchall term "intestinal flu," although they are not caused by the influenza virus. In fact, most viral gastroenteritis is caused by water or food contaminated by Norwalk virus or by rotavirus, and epidemics often occur among two vulnerable populations, the very young in day-care centers and the elderly living in nursing homes.

Diarrhea caused by bacteria—infectious gastroenteritis—often comes from the eating of contaminated food, usually the result of poor food-handling practices, and can involve any of a number of organisms, the most common being campylobacter, salmonella, and many variant forms of *Escherichia coli* (*E. coli*). Store-bought food such as eggs and chicken can also be contaminated. In the late 1990s, an increasing incidence of hemorrhagic *E. coli* from foods contaminated at processing or packaging facilities has been occurring, resulting in epidemics of illness and even death.

Diarrhea caused by parasitic infection is the least prevalent of the common diarrheas in the United States. Most often it is caused by *Giardia lamblia*, found in the water of contaminated streams, lakes or wells, or in swimming pools that use these sources.

These diarrheal illnesses are usually self-limiting, resolving in three to seven days. If diarrhea persists for longer than that, a doctor needs to look for long-term causes, including inflammatory bowel disease. The doctor will want to know if the diarrhea occurs at night or in the early morning. Diarrhea that awakens a person hints at organic disease rather than a functional problem, such as irritable bowel syndrome. The doctor will also want to know if the diarrhea is bloody or contains mucus or pus. While ulcerative colitis is characterized by bloody and mucus- or pus-streaked diarrhea, this condition is less prevalent in Crohn disease. Occasionally an individual will have relatively normal stools, accompanied by bleeding.

Pain

How much abdominal pain an individual has, as well as the "quality" of the pain, is also an important indicator for a doctor taking a medical history if inflammatory bowel disease is suspected. Pain is dependent on where within the bowel the disease is located, and is often an indication of the severity of the disease.

For those with ulcerative colitis, the pain is usually crampy in nature and more apparent on the left side. This is logical, since the large intestine (the colon) descends on the left; the descending colon joins the sigmoid colon, which then joins the rectum. Ulcerative colitis is continuous inflammation that starts at the rectum and ends at some point in the colon (discussed later in subtypes of ulcerative colitis). Often, a bowel movement leads to relief or at least a lessening of the pain.

Those who suffer from Crohn disease often have more persistent pain, which is frequently less crampy and sharper. The pain is usually most apparent around the navel, and can signal a bowel obstruction or an inflammatory mass. Crohn disease pain also often occurs in the right lower quadrant of the abdomen. Either of these types of pain points to disease where it is most prevalent in those with Crohn disease, in the terminal ileum (the last few inches of the small intestine as it moves horizontally from left to right under the navel), which joins the initial section of the colon, the cecum, in the lower right quadrant.

The appendix also sits at this junction of the ileum and the cecum. Because of the pain and fever associated with Crohn disease, an incorrect diagnosis of appendicitis may be made, and some cases of Crohn disease have been identified after a healthy appendix was removed.

Those with Crohn disease may also feel the pain increase after eating. This is because the opening at the diseased portion of the small intestine may be so inflamed (and may also be thickened and scarred) that an obstruction is formed that makes it difficult for food to pass through.

Diarrhea, and sometimes even pain, can also be caused by a condition called irritable bowel syndrome. Sometimes mistakenly confused with inflammatory bowel disease, irritable bowel syndrome is a functional motility disorder of the gastrointestinal tract, while IBD is an organic inflammatory disease. (The term "motility" refers to the involuntary movement of smooth muscles, such as those in the intestinal tract.) Irritable bowel syndrome is a physiological reaction many people experience in relation to stress and anxiety; indeed, it is a condition often found in those with clinically diagnosed anxiety disorders. Confusion of irritable bowel syndrome with organic inflammatory bowel disease has led many to designate IBD as a psychosomatic problem for much of this century.

While it has been known for many years that anxiety, stress, and tension do not cause inflammatory bowel disease, we are coming to realize that, in any chronic illness, physical symptoms of a disease's flare-up often go hand-in-hand with exacerbation of psychological symptoms of stress. Today, however, it is known that this mind/body connection is complicated, and this matter will be discussed in detail in chapter 6.

Fever

Fever is the third classic symptom of inflammatory bowel disease. Both Crohn disease and ulcerative colitis are inflammatory conditions, which are often accompanied by fever. Some people suffer from a high fever, especially if the inflammation is acute or if there is an abscess (a pocket of infection, usually bacterial). Those with inflammatory bowel disease are prone to have abscesses form outside the bowel wall. These are usually the result of microperforations of the bowel wall, or fistulas.

More common is a low-grade fever. Adults may not even take their temperature and know they have a fever; they may merely be cranky, irritable, and lethargic. Sometimes, the fever comes during the day and breaks during the night, leading to "night sweats."

Other Important Signs and Symptoms

A number of extraintestinal manifestations of inflammatory bowel disease can appear, sometimes many months before any significant appearance of bowel symptoms. Some occur immediately before a flare-up of bowel inflammation. Even if they are not present at the time of a physical exam, the physician who suspects inflammatory bowel disease will ask about them in taking a patient's complete history.

These signs and symptoms include reddening and inflammation of the eyes, joint pains, and skin lesions. Sores inside the mouth, called aphthous ulcers, may also appear in those with either Crohn disease or ulcerative colitis. Children and teenagers with inflammatory bowel disease may show impairment in both growth and sexual maturation. Another symptom is weight loss over time, brought about by poor appetite because of pain and diarrhea. Malabsorption of nutrients may even lead to malnutrition, which can be determined through some of the laboratory tests discussed later in this chapter.

The Physical Exam

In addition to carrying out the routine aspects of a physical exam, the doctor who suspects inflammatory bowel disease will focus extra attention on two areas: the abdomen for tenderness and inflammatory mass and the anorectal area for a number of signs, as shown in figure 1.1.

The doctor will feel gently in the right lower quadrant of the abdomen to see if there is a palpable inflammatory mass. This mass, sometimes present in Crohn disease, is caused by current acute inflammation, usually at the ileum, as well as by a thickening of the intestinal wall and scar tissue developed from chronic or recurrent inflammation. There may also be a thickening of the mesentery, the fatty tissue that holds the intestines together.

The mass may include a number of "loops" of small intestine that are adhering to each other, and fistulas (inappropriate openings that connect the intestine with another organ or with itself) may occur within the loops.

The doctor will also feel along the path of the colon, up the right side, across under the diaphragm, and down the left side, searching for tender spots that signal areas of acute inflammation, which can occur either in ulcerative colitis or in Crohn disease of the colon.

While people who suffer from ulcerative colitis often have a normal anal exam, those with Crohn disease can show any one of a number of abnormalities, many of which are very painful. Among these are hemorrhoids; anal fissures (cracks in the lining of the anus, which are extraordinarily painful); thick, cauliflower-like mounds that are quite tender; false openings called sinus tracts, which often give off a discharge; and perianal abscesses, which also frequently drain. Women may have a fistula between the rectum and the vagina. Figure I.I shows an abnormal perianal region.

A doctor who suspects inflammatory bowel disease will perform a rectal exam, inserting a gloved and lubricated finger into the rectum. People with ulcerative colitis may have a subtle irregularity of the tissue lining the rectum that signals ulceration. Those with Crohn disease may have a severely narrowed anorectum, which the doctor cannot pass a finger through. Blood may be detected during the exam.

Lab Tests

A number of laboratory tests should be taken to add evidence for a diagnosis of inflammatory bowel disease.

As part of the rectal exam, the doctor will test to see if there is

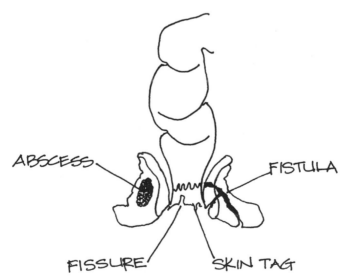

FIG. I.I Perianal irregularities common in Crohn disease.

any blood on the stool smear on the glove (called occult blood), which reveals bleeding in the intestinal tract.

Blood drawn from a vein in the arm will be subjected to many tests. Both the white blood count and the erythrocyte (red blood cell) sedimentation rate may be elevated, signaling an inflammatory process somewhere in the body. The hemoglobin in the red cells as well as the hematocrit (the ratio of red blood cells to whole blood) may be lower than normal, indicating anemia, which is due to malabsorption of iron, excessive bleeding, or chronic illness.

Others that might be performed include liver function tests and tests to measure the absorption of important nutrients. A stool sample might be tested in an effort to rule out bacterial or parasitic causes of the diarrhea, although this is not 100 percent accurate.

Diagnostic Procedures

The most common diagnostic procedures performed when inflammatory bowel disease is suspected are the sigmoidoscopy, colonoscopy, two barium X-ray series (the barium enema and the upper-GI series with small bowel follow-through), and an endoscopic exam of the esophagus and stomach, which is done with an endoscope that passes through the mouth.

Sigmoidoscopy

Sigmoidoscopy is occasionally performed with a short, rigid scope, but far more frequently with a sixty-centimeter flexible scope. Sigmoidoscopy is almost always conducted in a doctor's office or a health clinic.

Most sigmoidoscopy is performed with one of the flexible fiber-optic tubes. The tube contains a light source and a camera lens. The doctor, looking for irregularities, inserts the sigmoidoscope into the anus, then moves it up through the rectum if a thirty-centimeter scope is being used (beyond if it is the sixty-centimeter scope) into the descending colon.

In addition to ulceration, signs of ulcerative colitis include a loss of "normal vascularity" to the lining of the bowel (excessive blood flow due to inflammation), a granular texture to the bowel lining (granularity), and easy bruising (friability). Changes to the appearance of the bowel wall are continuous in ulcerative colitis, starting in the rectum and moving up through the colon. They can stop at any point.

In Crohn disease with active involvement of the colon, changes to the colon wall appear as ulcerations that can run from tiny and shallow to large and deep, as well as erosions in the colon lining. "Skip areas" of healthy tissue often appear between areas of diseased tissue. Deep linear ulcerations alternating with areas of healing mucosa cause the classic "cobblestone" pattern of Crohn colitis.

The procedure takes between five and twenty minutes. Some local discomfort may occur, and those with active inflammatory bowel disease may have some pain. Preparation for the procedure is one to two enemas approximately one hour before the exam.

Colonoscopy

Colonoscopy, a more thorough examination of the large intestine, allows visualization of the entire colon and of the terminal ileum, which is helpful in distinguishing Crohn disease from ulcerative colitis. A colonoscope is longer than a sigmoidoscope. Electronic imaging making use of microchips and screen projection is replacing the older fiber-optic technology. Medications given before the examination make it quite tolerable. However, because of the medication, people typically will need to take a day off from work and will require a ride home after the procedure.

For a complete colonoscopy, which is used for cancer screening as well as for diagnosing inflammatory bowel disease, a more complete bowel cleansing, beginning the day before the procedure, is necessary. A number of different preparations can be prescribed for bowel cleansing; doctors have preferences, and if you need to undergo a bowel cleansing for a colonoscopy or for bowel surgery, don't assume that you should use a preparation you have used in the past with a different doctor.

Barium Enema

In this procedure, barium is inserted into the rectum and colon through a tube placed in the rectum, and a series of X rays is taken. Standard X rays do not distinguish soft tissues such as the intestinal tract very well, especially the lining of the bowel, which must be seen clearly if the right diagnosis is to be made. Because of this, barium is used as a contrast agent. Barium allows a radiologist and a gastroenterologist (a physician who specializes in diseases of the intestinal tract, liver, and other organs of the abdomen) to more easily detect areas of disease by the way the barium appears on the X ray.

Enough barium is inserted to fill the entire colon, and some usually moves slightly beyond the ileocecal valve into the ileum. This often allows for a good visualization of Crohn disease of the ileum. A barium enema is often a definitive test in making the diagnosis of Crohn disease.

As with the colonoscopy, a thorough purging and cleansing of the bowel is necessary to eliminate all stool before the exam.

Upper-GI X Ray with Small Bowel Follow-Through

In the other barium study used to diagnose Crohn disease and to pinpoint its location and the severity of tissue damage, barium is swallowed and time is allowed to pass while the barium coats the lining of the esophagus, the stomach, and the entire small intestine. Again, a series of X rays is taken.

No bowel preparation is needed for this study; an individual need only refrain from eating or drinking for about ten hours before the exam.

The radiologist uses a compression paddle to compress the abdomen and separate the loops of small intestine enough so that the X rays will show clearly whether the final loops of the terminal ileum are narrowed. If this is the case, a narrow strand of barium—a string sign—will be apparent where the small intestine ends, just before it spreads out again in the colon.

The Nine Varieties of Inflammatory Bowel Disease

If a diagnosis of either Crohn disease or ulcerative colitis is made, a subtype name will often be given. Various systems are used to categorize patients and their diseases. These categories are all somewhat arbitrary. Some people find them useful, while others do not. Whatever the categorization scheme, the various subtypes of Crohn disease or ulcerative colitis should not be thought of as separate diseases but rather as variations on a theme.

The subtypes of Crohn disease and ulcerative colitis given here are used to define the location of disease within the intestinal system. The types of disease have different symptoms and different treatment regimens; these will be discussed in later chapters.

Ulcerative Colitis: Four Categories

In those with ulcerative colitis, a distinct portion of the colon is diseased. Disease starts at the rectum and moves "up" the colon to involve more of the organ. In some individuals, disease never moves from the area that is affected when a diagnosis is made; in others, the disease progresses over time, involving more of the colon. The four subtypes are ulcerative proctitis, proctosigmoiditis, left-sided colitis, and pancolitis.

Ulcerative Proctitis

Ulcerative proctitis is limited to the rectum. Symptoms usually include diarrhea (although some individuals suffer from constipation), bloody stool, and a sense of urgency to empty the bowel, as well as pain in the rectal area (called tenesmus) (fig. 1.2).

Proctosigmoiditis

Proctosigmoiditis affects the rectum and sigmoid colon—the first fifteen to fifty centimeters or so of the left colon above the rectum. Symptoms are diarrhea, bloody stool, cramps, and tenesmus. Moderate pain (persistent and crampy) often occurs on the left side of the abdomen when the disease is active.

Left-sided Colitis

Left-sided colitis involves the entire left or descending colon, from the rectum to the splenic flexure, where the colon bends near the spleen and begins to run across the upper abdomen. Symptoms include diarrhea, bleeding, weight loss, and loss of

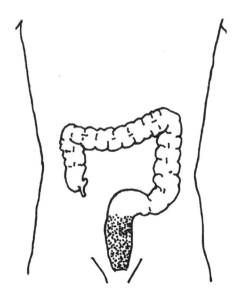

FIG. 1.2 Ulcerative proctitis.

appetite. Severe pain sometimes occurs on the left side of the abdomen (fig. 1.3).

Pancolitis

Pancolitis is colitis that affects the entire colon. Although the term may appear to be describing a severe form of colitis, in truth the severity of the illness is not determined by the amount of colon involved. An individual's symptoms may be mild, moderate, or severe whether the entire colon or only the rectum is involved. The significance of the diagnosis of pancolitis relates to the treatment options available. While ulcerative proctitis or left-sided colitis can be treated with local agents, including steroid and other enemas and foams, pancolitis must be treated with systemic medications, taken orally, that allow active agents to reach the entire colon (fig. 1.4).

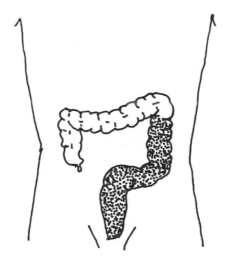

FIG. 1.3 Left-sided ulcerative colitis.

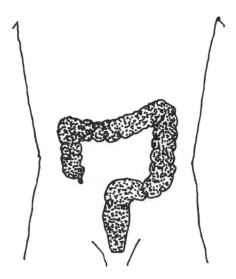

FIG. 1.4 Pancolitis.

Crohn Disease: Five Categories

While Crohn disease lesions can appear anywhere in the gastrointestinal tract, from the mouth to the anus, lesions in the mouth or esophogus rarely appear unless disease also occurs farther down in the gastrointestinal system. The five subtypes of Crohn disease (not in order of frequency of occurence) are gastroduodenal Crohn disease, jejunoileitis, ileitis, ileocolitis, and Crohn colitis (also called granulomatous colitis).

Gastroduodenal Crohn Disease

Gastroduodenal Crohn disease affects the stomach and the duodenum (the beginning of the small intestine). This condition is often diagnosed initially as ulcer disease, with the correct diagnosis not being made until after treatment for ulcers has been unsuccessful or until Crohn disease has been diagnosed in another part of the intestinal tract. Symptoms include loss of appetite and weight loss, nausea, pain in the upper middle of the abdomen, and vomiting.

Jejunoileitis

Jejunoileitis is Crohn disease of the jejunum, the largest part of the small intestine, which is located between the duodenum and the ileum. The major symptom is mild-to-intense abdominal pain and cramps after meals. Diarrhea sometimes occurs, and malabsorption of the nutrients normally absorbed in this region can lead to weight loss and malnutrition. (Intestinal absorption of nutrients will be discussed in detail in chapter 2.) Fistulas may form and link one diseased area to other loops of bowel or to other organs.

Ileitis

Ileitis affects the ileum, the last part of the small intestine. The main symptoms are diarrhea and cramping or pain in the right-lower and lower-middle part of the abdomen, especially after meals. Malabsorption of vitamin B_{12} can lead to peripheral neuropathy (tingling fingers or toes), and folate deficiency can hinder red blood cell development. Fistulas sometimes occur, as do obstructions, and inflammatory mass is sometimes apparent in the right lower abdomen.

Ileocolitis

Ileocolitis is the most common variety of Crohn disease. As the name suggests, it affects the ileum and the colon. Often the diseased areas of the ileum and colon are contiguous and involve the ileocecal valve, which sits at the junction of the ileum and the cecum—the first section of the colon—and keeps the waste contents of the colon from backflushing into the small intestine. Sometimes areas of the colon not close to the ileum are also involved. Symptoms are essentially the same as the ones for ileitis. Weight loss is also common.

Crohn Colitis (Granulomatous Colitis)

Crohn colitis affects only the colon. Symptoms are diarrhea, rectal bleeding, and pain. The condition is often difficult to differentiate from ulcerative colitis (misdiagnosis occurs up to 20 percent of the time). However, the presence of disease around the anus, including fistulas and abscesses, leads to a diagnosis of Crohn colitis rather than ulcerative colitis. Other features that should help distinguish Crohn colitis from ulcerative colitis include rectal sparing (no disease in the rectum), skip lesions (an area of disease followed by an area of healthy tissue, then by another area of disease), and apthous ulcers. Extraintestinal symptoms such as joint pain and skin lesions are more common with this subtype of Crohn disease than with others.

Another Crohn Disease Subtyping System

Some doctors also distinguish subtypes of Crohn disease as inflammatory, fistulizing, and obstructing. This classification scheme is not always precise, since obstructing disease often also has characteristics of inflammation and vice versa. The classification refers to the predominant symptoms—how the disease primarily presents itself. However, an individual may have a bowel obstruction and/or inflammatory mass and/or one or more fistulas. Fistulas are the most difficult complication of Crohn disease; many are refractory to medical treatment, and surgical correction often does not stop other fistulas from occurring.

Figure 1.5 shows the intestinal complications of Crohn disease: widespread inflammation, fistula, stricture, and abscess.

The Importance of Getting the Right Diagnosis

Appropriate diagnosis is necessary for a number of reasons.

First, it is important to rule out a self-limiting gastrointestinal illness caused by a virus, bacterium, or parasite. There is no need

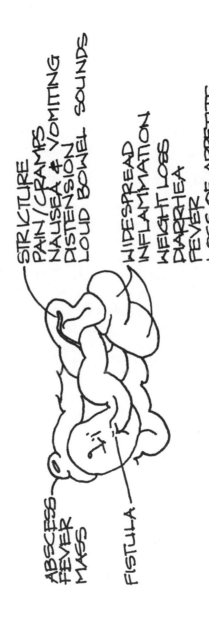

FIG. 1.5 Small-bowel complications of Crohn disease.

to begin someone on a regimen of long-term and sometimes toxic medical therapy for a short-term illness.

Second, it is inappropriate to treat infectious diseases with anti-inflammatory drugs or steroids, two of the most powerful groups of medications used for inflammatory bowel disease. These drugs do nothing for an infectious disease, and they are potentially toxic. Their toxicity is acceptable only because they are so effective when used properly in treatment.

Third, the diagnosis of inflammatory bowel disease carries a number of long-term implications. In addition to the medical treatment regimen itself, there is a need for heightened screening for intestinal cancer because of the statistically increased risk. Also, the diagnosis may affect an individual's ability to purchase medical, disability, and even life insurance.

Fourth, a number of surgical options can be taken to treat persistent and nonresponsive cases of inflammatory bowel disease. Misdiagnosis could lead to inappropriate surgery.

Finally, as researchers get closer to discovering both the causes of these diseases and the different ways in which they affect cells, the importance of proper diagnosis increases. Throughout the twentieth century, treatment of these diseases has been essentially a matter of trial and error. Even today, it is not known why certain medications have the effects they do on Crohn disease and ulcerative colitis.

For example, in late 1998, the Food and Drug Administration approved infliximab, the first medication specifically for Crohn disease. Infliximab (sold under the trade name Remicade) is a genetically engineered substance that has no effect on ulcerative colitis. In Crohn disease, it helps heal fistulas that have been unresponsive to other treatment, and can bring about clinical remission of inflammatory symptoms.

A number of other medications that may work on one or both of the inflammatory bowel diseases are still in the clinical trial stage.

The Value of a Second Opinion

Because the correct diagnosis of inflammatory bowel disease is so important, and because the disease presents so many variations and nuances, it may be wise for people to get a second opinion in any case where the diagnosis is not absolutely clear-cut.

This is especially true if the original diagnosis is made by an internist or family practitioner who does not see many new cases of Crohn disease or ulcerative colitis in the course of a year. Whenever possible, an individual should have a complete examination performed by a gastroenterologist, who sees patients with these diseases on a daily basis.

2. How the Healthy Digestive System Works

The digestive system is a series of hollow, tubular structures running from the mouth to the anus. It includes the esophagus, stomach, small intestine, and large intestine. As food travels through this system, it is broken down into small units that are absorbed by the lining cells of the intestine and transported into the bloodstream.

If the digestive system is to function properly, it must work in coordination with other internal organs: the liver, which produces bile; the gallbladder, which stores bile; and the pancreas, which produces digestive enzymes.

Digestion transforms fats into fatty acids and glycerol, proteins into amino acids, and carbohydrates into simple sugars, all to be used by the body as energy or as chemical building blocks. If a person overeats, all of the nutrients not used as energy or for maintaining body structure and function can be converted into body fat.

Digestive enzymes, found mostly in the liver and the pancreas, are chemicals manufactured in the body that help break down food into its nutrient components.

The energy we get from food is measured in calories, a unit that refers to the amount of heat necessary to raise one gram of water one degree centigrade. Saying that a portion of food has 250 calories means that when the food is digested and absorbed, it provides 250 calories' worth of energy that the body can use.

The number of calories an individual needs to maintain daily activity depends on the person's size, level of physical activity, and health. When inflammation is present, heat is being generated and more calories are being used; calories are also being burned by fever. Hence, fighting inflammatory bowel disease actually requires a higher caloric intake than a healthy person needs; this will be discussed in more detail in chapter 4.

Caloric intake should not be confused with nutrition. It is possible for a person to take in enough calories and still be malnourished. That can happen when the nutrients necessary for proper nourishment are not fully absorbed or when the calories are taken in from nonnutritive items. For instance, alcohol has a lot of calories but little nutritional value, which is why alcoholics can be simultaneously overweight and malnourished. In the case of an individual with inflammatory bowel disease, malabsorption and malnourishment are potential problems, as we will see in chapter 3.

From the Top: The Mouth and Esophagus

Digestion begins in the mouth, when food is chewed to a mushy consistency and is then propelled down the esophagus into the stomach by peristalsis, a series of wave-like motions. Peristalsis continues to push the food through the entire digestive system until the waste exits at the anus.

In the mouth, food is mixed with saliva created by the salivary glands and begins to be broken down by ptyalin, the salivary enzyme that breaks down carbohydrates into simple sugars. Food passes from the mouth down the esophagus. At the end of the esophagus is a valve-like muscle (the lower esophageal sphincter), which allows food to pass from the esophagus to the stomach but normally does not allow food to go back up into the esophagus.

Preabsorption: The Stomach

Inside the stomach, food begins to be broken down into more discrete nutritional components by means of both muscular action and stomach juices. The stomach wall has a number of muscle layers that cause the stomach to churn and break food into smaller and smaller pieces that can be acted upon by the stomach juices.

The stomach has several functions. It provides a storage space where food can be digested over time. It acts like a mechanical mixer, combining the food with stomach juices and furthering digestion. It releases food into the small intestine in portions small enough to be acted on efficiently.

Through a series of muscular contractions, the semiliquid substance known as chyme is forced out of the stomach through the pyloric canal into the upper portion of the small intestine (small bowel) called the duodenum. Later, the very small particles of the more solid material are also pushed into the duodenum.

Finally, the stomach produces useful substances such as intrinsic factor, which are necessary for the absorption of vitamin B_{12}. The main ingredient of these stomach juices is pepsin, an enzyme that begins the digestion of food. Hydrochloric acid in the stomach creates an environment in which pepsin can work. However, only a small bit of nutrient absorption occurs in the stomach itself, which mostly performs a preabsorption function, turning the mass of food into chyme.

From Food to Fuel: The Small Intestine

Three parts of the small intestine—the duodenum, the jejunum, and the ileum—conduct some of the absorptive function. The duodenum is the shortest part; the jejunum, the middle portion, is the longest; and the ileum is also relatively short. In an adult, the entire small intestine can run from twelve to eighteen feet, depending on its muscle tone.

Food continues to churn in the duodenum. In addition, the stomach acids are neutralized there. Bile ducts from both the gallbladder and the liver also feed bile into the duodenum. Bile is produced continuously in the liver and fed into the duodenum as needed to help absorb fats. Excess bile is stored in the gallbladder for use when there is more fat than can be absorbed by the bile produced by the liver at any one time.

Most digestion takes place in the jejunum. Carbohydrates are broken down into simple sugars, proteins are broken down into amino acids, and fats are broken down into fatty acids. Bile acids render fat molecules soluble in water. All of these nutrients, as well as vitamins, minerals, water, and electrolytes such as calcium and salt, are absorbed through the walls of the small intestine into the bloodstream.

At the ileum, vitamin B_{12}, the final nutrient to be extracted from food, is absorbed. The food remnants then pass through the ileocecal valve into the colon.

Figure 2.1 depicts the major sections of the gastrointestinal tract, and shows how essential nutrients are absorbed from the small intestine.

Eliminating Waste: The Colon

No absorption of nutrients takes place in the colon; the colon's main function is to reabsorb water from the waste material, store the solid waste, and eliminate it through the voluntary muscles at the anus.

The colon is highly efficient. Almost all the water that enters a healthy person's colon every day is reabsorbed, with only about 0.1 of one quart remaining in the waste as it passes through the colon's five sections—the right (cecum and ascending colon); the transverse (cross) colon; the left (descending) colon; the sigmoid colon; and the rectum, approximately the last fifteen centimeters of the colon. From the rectum, the waste passes out the anus.

The Supporting Cast: Liver, Gallbladder, and Pancreas

The liver performs many important functions. In addition to producing bile, the liver stores glycogen, a complex carbohydrate, and converts it into glucose (sugar) for release

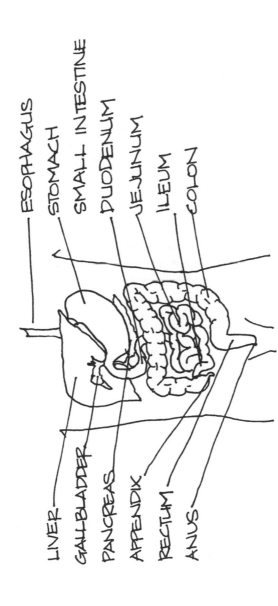

FIG. 2.1 Gastrointestinal tract, including where nutrients are absorbed. Iron, fat, sugars, amino acids, and folic acid are absorbed into the duodenum. Vitamins A, D, E, and K, Vitamin C, niacin, and thiamin are absorbed into the jejunum. Vitamin B[12] and bile salts are absorbed into the ileum.

into the bloodstream when the blood sugar level falls. Glycogen is deposited in the liver when the blood sugar level is high. This organ also serves as a regulator, determining how much of various kinds of nutrients is sent throughout the body. In addition, the liver metabolizes a number of medications, converting them into the most useful chemical form for treating various illnesses.

The gallbladder is not an essential organ, serving only to store bile produced by the liver that is not being used immediately. It can be removed with minimal consequence.

The pancreas is essential. It produces pancreatic enzymes, which are secreted through the pancreatic ducts into the duodenum and assist in digestion of fats and proteins. The pancreas also produces the hormones insulin and glucagon, which are released directly into the bloodstream and regulate the metabolism of glucose (sugar), amino acids, fatty acids, and glycogen in the liver and other tissues.

When the digestive system is healthy, the transformation of food into energy and waste is automatic. But when the digestive system is damaged by inflammatory bowel disease, any or all of its various components can malfunction, leading to malabsorption, malnutrition, and severe damage to the quality of life.

3. How and Why the Digestive System Malfunctions in People with Crohn Disease or Ulcerative Colitis

The major pathology of the intestinal tract in a person with Crohn disease or ulcerative colitis is chronic inflammation. Inflammation is a natural response when the body's immune system "attacks" a foreign entity (antigen). Inflammation is characterized by four conditions: heat, redness, pain and swelling. The antigen can be viral, bacterial, parasitic, or chemical; it can be a foreign physical object such as a wood splinter or foreign tissue such as a transplanted organ. But with Crohn disease or ulcerative colitis, there is no obvious immediate antigen at hand. The immune response seems inappropriate; the body creates inflammation with no reason to do so.

In cases of Crohn disease or ulcerative colitis, the inflammation occurs in the inside of the gastrointestinal tract. The inflammatory process also causes damage to the cellular structure of the intestine.

The intestine's lining, the mucosa, is thin; inflammation damages it and can break the protective barrier it forms. When ulcerations develop, intestinal tissue is exposed to the harmful effects of intestinal contents, as well as to enzymes released by inflammatory cells.

In ulcerative colitis, the inflammation only affects the mucosa. In Crohn disease, however, the inflammation can go through the mucosa and involve the full thickness of the bowel wall. The nature of tissue involvement helps the gastroenterologist categorize the Crohn disease as either the inflammatory form (in which the inflammation may cause an inflammatory mass), the obstructing form (in which the inflammation on the inside of the intestine actually causes the intestinal opening to close off; scar tissue from healing inflammation can also close it off), or the fistulizing form (where loops of bowel become connected by a fistula that runs from the inside of one loop to the inside of another).

Depending on where in the gastrointestinal tract the inflammation occurs, effects include malabsorption of nutrients, bleeding, diarrhea, fever, and pain.

Inflammation usually has a cause, or precipitator. But researchers have not yet been able to find a specific precipitator for Crohn disease or ulcerative colitis. They can see the primary sign of the malfunction within the gastrointestinal system (the inflammation) and the secondary symptoms (the bleeding, diarrhea, pain, fatigue, and fever). How and why the malfunction occurs is still a mystery.

To date, the best hypothesis can be shown in this equation: genetic factor(s) + environmental precipitator(s) = inappropriate inflammatory response.

Researchers today are focusing on a number of key questions about the inflammatory process. They are trying to determine not only how, but, more important, why the inappropriate inflammatory response occurs in those with Crohn disease and ulcerative colitis. Some of the key questions are: What triggers the immune system response? What is the genetic component? Is there an inflammatory bowel disease gene? What is the effect of environmental factors such as diet, water, and chemicals? What kind of precipitating incidents lead to an initial bout of either Crohn disease or ulcerative colitis? Do other precipitating incidents cause flare-ups?

A Few Statistics

Inflammatory bowel disease appears to be an affliction primarily of those living in Western, industrialized societies.

Crohn disease and ulcerative colitis are rarely diagnosed in less developed countries. Epidemiologists—people who study statistical information about health and illness—have found an inverse relationship between IBD and the prevalence of infectious diarrheas, those caused by bacteria and parasites.

Whether inflammatory bowel disease does not exist in certain areas or whether the high incidence of acute infectious gastrointestinal illnesses simply masks the presence of the more chronic conditions is unclear. Unfortunately, in less developed parts of the world few funds are available to do extensive diagnostic testing of people suffering from diarrhea; their symptoms are treated, and they get better or die. Epidemiologists wonder whether the reason for this correlation has to do with something in the environments of industrialized societies, or whether underlying cases of inflammatory bowel disease are simply not diagnosed in less developed countries.

One group of researchers at the University of Iowa theorized that the preponderance of IBD in the industrialized world may, indeed, be the result of the eradication of certain parasites called helminths. Helminths are worms that live in the intestinal tracts of many animals and of people who live in regions of the world without sanitary sewer facilities. Working on the notion that all creatures provide some benefit to their environment, these researchers were interested in the question of whether the eradication of helminths over the last few centuries resulting from better sanitation facilities in the Western world could have had an unintended consequence—an increase in the incidence of autoimmune diseases such as IBD, multiple sclerosis, rheumatoid arthritis, and lupus. They gave six people suffering from an acute flare-up of IBD a drink containing the eggs of a half-inch-long helminth commonly found in pig intestines, but which cannot reproduce in the human intestine. Five went into remission; the sixth improved. There were no side effects. All relapsed after the worms left their systems.

Even if the eradication of helminths in the intestines of people living in industrialized countries is part of the reason for

IBD's prevalence in those places, the following statistics are still somewhat difficult to interpret.

Inflammatory bowel disease is most prevalent in the United States, the United Kingdom, Scandinavia, and Western Europe. Within those countries, rates are about five times higher in the Jewish population than in the general population. Among the Jewish population in Israel, people of European or American background have a much higher rate of inflammatory bowel disease than those of Asian, North African, or Middle Eastern background.

Asians have little inflammatory bowel disease, except in Japan, where the rates have been rising steadily since the country began to industrialize after the Second World War.

There is little inflammatory bowel disease among Africans, although African Americans do experience IBD, and, among African American women aged twenty to forty, the rate of disease is almost equal to that in the population of white women the same age.

While difficult to interpret, these statistics continue to lead researchers to think that a "Western diet," which is high in animal fats and protein and relatively low in fruits, vegetables, and fiber, plays some part in the development of Crohn disease and ulcerative colitis. However, diet cannot, strictly speaking, be considered a "cause," since studies have not found that those within the population at large whose intake of protein and animal fat is higher than normal have an increased incidence of inflammatory bowel disease. And, despite the fact that more Americans are eating healthier diets today than was so a generation ago, the incidence of Crohn disease continues to rise.

Nor can environmental factors be specifically singled out as "causes" of inflammatory bowel disease. Those who live in cities, suburbs, and rural areas are equally likely to suffer from Crohn disease or ulcerative colitis. No worker group has a high incidence of inflammatory bowel disease and can thus point to a particular workplace hazard. Nor is there any one substance that has been shown to cause "clusters" of inflammatory bowel disease cases in neighborhoods, as has been the case with certain cancers.

The Genetic Front

Statistics are helpful in looking at familial patterns of inflammatory bowel disease. Crohn disease and ulcerative colitis are "familial" or "complex" genetic diseases, as opposed to "simple" genetic diseases.

In simple genetic diseases such as sickle cell disease or cystic fibrosis, a person who inherits a copy of the defective gene from each parent is certain to get the disease. In Crohn disease or ulcerative colitis, this is not the case. In fact, 85–90 percent of people with Crohn disease or ulcerative colitis have no relatives with either disease. At the same time, because there are fewer than one million Americans who live with inflammatory bowel disease, the 10–15 percent multiple incidence in families means that the risk of the disease is statistically higher when a family member has IBD than when the disease is not present.

No typical pattern in family histories points to the diseases following the laws of Mendelian genetics. Thus, there is no way to predict the probability of a particular couple producing a child who will develop IBD.

Ample evidence of a genetic factor exists, however. First, some populations that bred closely within their communities for many generations (Eastern European Jews, for instance) have a higher incidence of inflammatory bowel diseases than other groups. Second, in the case of Crohn disease, both the disease location (small intestine, colon, or both) and the clinical subtype (fistulas, mass, or stricture/obstruction) are similar in family members who have the disease.

Scientists are beginning to home in on the genetic link. A number of genes and gene regions on six different chromosomes (1p, 3, 6, 7, 12, and 16) are associated with the development of

Crohn disease. In addition, genetics plays a role in the function of the body's immune system.

And evidence indicates that each different form of Crohn disease and ulcerative colitis has its own particular disease process, with varying symptoms, and its own genetic factors. This may include one dominant gene, two recessive genes, or a host of genes acting together.

The Immunology Contribution

AIDS research has furthered our understanding of how the immune system works and also of how it doesn't work properly in diseases such as Crohn disease and ulcerative colitis. Inflammatory bowel disease is the result of abnormal control of the immune response to environmental triggers. These triggers may include the bacteria that occur naturally in a person's own gastrointestinal tract.

The immune system is responsible for manufacturing cells that recognize and destroy antigens that invade the body. These cells include lymphocytes, monocytes, granulocytes, mast cells, and macrophages.

Lymphocytes are the most prevalent player in the immune response. They produce T cells, so called because they are produced in the thymus gland. One of these types of T cells, TH1 cells, along with macrophages, attack the offending antigen, promoting inflammation by producing three proinflammation chemicals, interleukin-1 (IL-1), IL-2, and tumor necrosis factor-alpha (TNF-alpha). TH2 cells, on the other hand, produce the anti-inflammatory chemicals IL-4, IL-10, transforming growth factor-beta (TGF-beta), and IL-1 receptor antagonists (IL-1ra), which slow down the inflammatory response after the antigen has been destroyed.

In the healthy intestine, invading bacteria are recognized as antigens and responded to immunologically, while those normally there are left alone. Between one billion and one trillion normal intestinal bacteria (enteric microflora) exist in every gram of intestinal content. The healthy intestine is "tolerant" of enteric microflora.

However, immunologic evidence indicates that in the intestines of those with IBD, some of this tolerance is lost. TH1 cells turn on the immune system in response to the normal enteric microflora, and the TH2 cells, for some reason, do not turn the response off. This causes an inappropriate inflammatory response and the attendant symptoms. Why most people's intestines display tolerance and a few people's do not remains a mystery.

Recent evidence also indicates that some inflammatory bowel disease may be a heightened immunologic response to seasonal allergies.

4. Living with the Condition

Crohn disease and ulcerative colitis are "bowel" diseases. But they can also affect many other parts of the body, directly or indirectly. In addition, a number of psychosocial effects are coincident to the diseases, involving issues such as self-image, feelings about chronic illness, and fears of other ailments, including colo-rectal cancer, inflammatory bowel disease-related arthritis, and osteoporosis, all of which will be discussed in detail.

People who live with inflammatory bowel disease are burdened by many questions. Will I always be sick? Will I be in constant pain? Will I forever be spending so much time seeing doctors? Will I die young? Will I become disabled so that I can't work? Will I ever get off high doses of medication? Will I be able to maintain my insurance?

This chapter takes a look at the lifelong effects of Crohn disease and ulcerative colitis and their impact on the quality of life. We'll discuss flare-ups of disease, nutrition, and the host of potential nonintestinal complications, as well as special situations such as the appearance of the diseases in children, effects on those of childbearing age, and Crohn disease and ulcerative colitis in the elderly.

A Lifelong Ailment

Although Crohn disease and ulcerative colitis are chronic, they are characterized by periods of remission that last for varying amounts of time, interrupted by flare-ups, when symptoms of the disease become more evident.

Each individual's pattern of symptoms is different, and conscientious doctors treat the symptoms, not the laboratory or radiological evidence. Individuals differ in their ways of coping with chronic illness, their tolerances to pain, and their ability to live with the uncertainty that comes with inflammatory bowel disease. Individuals who live with IBD also have varying degrees of support systems, made up of family, friends, work associates, and religious cocongregants.

Disease severity can be measured both objectively and subjectively. Because these diseases behave so erratically, the objective clinical signs do not always match up directly with the patient's subjective feeling of well-being or with the doctor's subjective view of the patient's condition. One individual with disease that looks severe when seen on radiological examination may have the ability to lead a relatively normal life, while another person with little objective evidence of disease may find the condition totally debilitating.

Pain, fatigue, fever, chills, vomiting, and diarrhea come and go, sometimes in waves and sometimes in sharp bursts. Some individuals try to "ride it out" between regular periodic visits to see the gastroenterologist who provides their care. Others lead lives seemingly controlled by the disease, seeing their doctor with each change of symptom.

Most individuals who live with inflammatory bowel disease seek some middle ground. They try to gauge for themselves what is a realistic "baseline" of discomfort and disruption that their disease causes, and seek medical advice when there are real changes from this baseline. Flare-ups caught early can often be treated more easily, although not always. By the time symptoms change, the inflammatory process is sometimes so far along that it is difficult to beat back.

When an individual with Crohn disease or ulcerative colitis is in the doctor's office, whether for a regular visit or for an urgent visit due to a specific change in symptoms, the examination has several components. The doctor does the following:

1. Asks a series of questions to get at the symptom pattern since the last visit. Asks about recent changes in signs and symptoms.

2. Checks vital signs such as blood pressure, temperature, and weight.

3. Performs a physical exam of the abdomen, gently palpating to feel for inflammatory mass, areas of tenderness, bloating, and possible changes in other internal organs such as the liver and spleen. May also perform a rectal exam.

4. Visually assesses the individual's general well-being.

5. Listens to and watches the individual closely for clues as to psychological state.

6. Possibly takes a blood sample for analysis.

By conducting this examination, the doctor can rank an individual's symptoms according to a well-defined disease index and characterize the symptoms as mild, moderate, or severe. Some individuals are never in a total remission, always having mild symptoms, while others can remain symptom free for years.

A sigmoidoscopy should not be part of a routine office visit. There is really no reason why a doctor needs to visualize the disease regularly. A sigmoidoscopy is, however, useful in dealing with a drastic change in the individual's condition, allowing the doctor to see whether the change is really due to a flare-up of inflammatory bowel disease or to some other illness.

An increase in symptoms is called a flare-up. Most flare-ups are transitory, lasting from a few weeks to a few months. Some resolve themselves with little or no treatment. Others respond well to the standard medication regimen, which will be discussed in chapter 5.

Flare-ups are distressing. They change all the normal rhythms of life. An individual experiencing a flare-up may have to take sick days from work or school, change social or family plans, or simply make sure to always be close to toilet facilities. Severe flare-ups can cause nutritional deficiency or dehydration from diarrhea, and can lead to hospitalization so that the condition can be brought under control.

Health care economists point out that the most expensive part of treatment for individuals with inflammatory bowel disease is hospitalization. Hospitalizations are not only costly in and of themselves, but mean lost work time for the ill individual as well as for family members. The increased risk of contracting a hospital-based illness such as a staph infection is also a factor. Treating flare-ups on an outpatient basis whenever possible is best for the ill individual and the family.

It is especially troubling when symptoms worsen and do not respond to medical treatment over time. Such disease is often characterized as "refractory" or even "intractable." Individuals with disease that is not responsive to the usual arsenal of medications may be referred to studies of experimental compounds, which are called clinical trials (these will be discussed in chapter 7). But for some, no treatment completely resolves the symptoms.

Some people find themselves debilitated to the point of being legally classified as "disabled" and therefore entitled to Social Security disability benefits and to benefits under private disability insurance, if they have such a policy. But with the host of recently approved, or experimental, medications, the vast majority of individuals who suffer flare-ups return to good health over time.

Now for the good news. The majority of people who live with inflammatory bowel disease are healthy more often than they are sick. The periods of remission are usually longer than the periods of flare-up. Few individuals need to stop working permanently because of IBD.

Nutritional Complications

Poor nutrition and even malnutrition are a constant threat to individuals with Crohn disease or ulcerative colitis for a number of reasons.

The disease creates a vicious cycle. Fever and diarrhea sap the appetite. Yet fever itself, by raising the metabolic rate, actually adds to the need for calories. Diarrhea can lead to dehydration and also to temporary lactose intolerance, the inability to digest milk sugars.

Dietary absorption is hindered, especially in those with Crohn disease of the small intestine and those who have bacterial overgrowth. Absorption occurs mostly in the the jejunum. People who suffer jejunoileitis, or who have had part of this region removed surgically because of the disease, suffer from poor nutrition and weight loss. Supplements contain sufficient nutritional components such that even a tiny fraction actually absorbed in other areas of the intestine is enough.

Many essential minerals are absorbed in the ileum. An individual with ileitis or ileocolitis, or whose ileum has been removed surgically, will suffer from malabsorption of these minerals. Many of the nutrients can be obtained only through supplements such as a multivitamin and regular intramuscular shots of vitamin B_{12}; again, these are so concentrated that enough is absorbed in other areas of the intestine.

Fat absorption is especially difficult because the ileum is where bile salts are reabsorbed. If they cannot be reabsorbed, they cannot be recycled, and that can lead to an inability to digest fats and a condition known as steatorrhea, symptoms of which are foul-smelling stools and cramping. Also, bile salts enter the colon, and, if they are malabsorbed, they cause secretion of water into the colon, leading to diarrhea; bile salts also alter the usually impermeable colon lining, causing it to absorb oxalate. Normal amounts of oxalate are excreted by the kidneys, but large amounts can crystallize into kidney stones (calcium oxalate.)

In those who are lactose intolerant, lactose ferments in the colon and creates cramping and more diarrhea. A dairy-free diet may be prescribed, which may in turn lead to more nutritional deficiency if calcium is lacking. Calcium deficiency over time can lead to loss of bone density, a condition known as osteoporosis. This can be especially dangerous to those being treated with corticosteriods such as prednisone. Prednisone use over time can lead to osteoporosis, even when the individual is consuming and absorbing calcium.

Another cause of nutritional complications is bacterial overgrowth. Normally, large amounts of bacteria inhabit the colon but not the small intestine. Up to half the mass of normal stool is bacteria. Usually, this bacteria is kept from moving back from the colon to the small intestine by the regular downward pressure of food moving through the intestines and by the ileocecal valve.

In many people with Crohn disease of the ileum, the ileocecal valve is not functioning properly, for any of a number of reasons. For example, in Crohn ileocolitis, the ileocecal valve itself is often diseased. A fistula may form between the small intestine and the colon, bypassing the ileocecal valve. During surgery to remove a badly diseased ileum, the diseased ileocecal valve is also removed.

In any of these cases, bacteria from the colon can back up into the small intestine, where they bind with bile salts, rendering the bile salts ineffective for fat digestion. Colonic bacteria can also create byproducts that are toxic to the intestinal lining, further affecting nutrient absorption.

In the case of ulcerative colitis, the nutritional issues are a little more simple to parse. The chronic diarrhea and pain create a loss of appetite, which means that at a time when more calories are needed the individual is taking in fewer.

Even some of the medications used to treat inflammatory bowel disease may exacerbate nutritional deficiency. Sulfasalazine reduces folic acid absorption. Steroids can lead to a loss of bone density. Some antibiotics used to treat bacterial overgrowth cause nausea and loss of appetite.

Treating Nutritional Deficiencies

Nutritional treatments for Crohn disease and ulcerative colitis have two main goals. The first is to increase the intake of calories, protein, vitamins, minerals, and trace elements to prevent nutritional deficiency. When there is active inflammation of the bowel, an individual requires 25 percent more protein than normal. The second is to create an eating pattern that minimizes stress on the diseased bowel. This usually means smaller, more frequent feedings. Many nutritional counselors suggest six half-sized meals, equally spaced, with the last one three or more hours before bedtime, because sleep slows down digestion.

Active Crohn disease sometimes narrows the small intestine so severely that larger food particles cannot fit through, thus creating an obstruction. In severe cases, the intestinal opening can close completely because of narrowing. An obstruction can be partial to complete. Obstructions are characterized by pain, nausea, and vomiting.

When a complete or nearly complete obstruction occurs, all oral feedings need to be stopped for a time. If the obstruction begins to resolve on its own, or with medication, within a matter of days, feedings begin with clear liquids such as broth, tea, and clear juices, progress to full liquids such as pulpy juices, and then to soft foods and a "normal" diet. It may be weeks or possibly even a few months before a normal diet is resumed. If the obstruction does not begin to resolve within a week or so, and the individual still can't tolerate oral feedings, the obstruction must be surgically removed or the individual must be put on a nutritionally complete intravenous feeding, called total parenteral nutrition (TPN), or liquid nutrition delivered directly to the stomach via a feeding tube, called total enteral nutrition (TEN), which we'll discuss in more detail shortly.

If an individual needs to be on a liquid diet for an extended period, a nutritional supplement can be added. These are canned formulas with the consistency of a milkshake; three to four cans a day provide enough nutrition. Some are lactose free, while others contain lactose. (Palatability of these products is only fair. Surgical residents in training who sometimes subsist on these supplements during long stretches in the operating room say that for maximum palatability, they drink plain vanilla, put it in the freezer for ten to twenty minutes, and add lots of chocolate syrup.)

It's also important to be wary of nutritional supplements that profess to boost the immune system.

Total Parenteral Nutrition: The Lifesaver Called TPN

In addition to providing periods of bowel rest while obstructions due to Crohn disease resolve, TPN is also used in a number of other situations:

To improve the nutritional health of a malnourished individual before bowel surgery. This greatly reduces the risk of postsurgical infections and other complications.

To provide lifetime feedings for an individual who has had so much small intestine removed because of Crohn disease that no nutrients from food taken orally are being absorbed, regardless of how much is eaten.

To provide periods of extended bowel rest for an individual with ulcerative colitis who is suffering a severe flare-up with intractable diarrhea. (This practice is controversial.)

While routine intravenous fluids administered through an arm contain sugar, water, salt, and small amounts of essential minerals, TPN contains all of the essential amino acids and higher concentrations of sugars, salts, minerals, vitamins, and trace elements needed for sustained nutritional health. A small vein would be terribly irritated by such a mixture. For that reason, TPN is administered through a catheter inserted into a major vein, usually the subclavian under the collarbone. This catheter can be surgically implanted for long-term use.

In fact, for long-term use, individuals can be taught how to administer their own TPN at home, while they sleep. With home TPN, an individual can lead a relatively normal life by day, without being tethered to any apparatus, or needing to be hospitalized, or even having to stay at home. Long courses of home TPN have changed the lives of many young people with Crohn disease or ulcerative colitis, allowing them to avoid extended hospital stays and many missed school days as they correct nutritional deficiency. Improving nutrition greatly improves the course of the disease and the quality of life of children with inflammatory bowel disease.

The only major downside to TPN is that it costs about a hundred thousand dollars per year. In addition, there are some issues having to do with maintaining the site where the infusion catheter is located.

What Is the Proper Diet for Those with Crohn Disease or Ulcerative Colitis?

Most doctors tell people with Crohn disease or ulcerative colitis that their diets should be "normal, as tolerated." One reason is that there is no conclusive evidence that any particular diet has any influence on the occurrence of a flare-up, or that any particular diet helps bring on reduction of symptoms any faster. A number of "special" diets are pitched by various nutrition authors (see the list of books about nutrition in appendix B).

Another reason is that dietary restrictions can create psychological distress for an individual who is already bearing the burden of chronic illness and has to confront issues of body image, frequency of bathroom use, and other special circumstances.

The most common dietary restrictions involve fiber, fat, and lactose. With the availability of synthetic lactase that can be taken in capsule form with milk products, there is usually no need for a lactose-free diet.

So-called elimination diets are used to systematically determine which foods, if any, create adverse effects. Elimination diets are usually attempted after an individual has been brought into a clinical remission. The person is started on a liquid diet, then "challenged" with one new food every day or every few days. Any food that causes ill effects is eliminated from the diet; those that don't are kept in. Some study evidence of elimination diets suggests that a number of individuals with IBD may be experiencing a hypersensitivity reaction to particular foods. But for most individuals with IBD, diets eliminating foods that have immediate ill effects have little or no bearing on whether an individual will stay in remission.

An interesting sidenote is that many people with Crohn disease or ulcerative colitis have found that avoiding caffeine helps, perhaps because caffeine increases gut motility.

The Question of Fiber

The term dietary fiber refers to the parts of plants that cannot be digested by humans. Dietary fiber is composed of many different components, which often cause opposing actions in the gut.

Low-fiber diets are often prescribed for individuals with Crohn disease or ulcerative colitis, the belief being that a low-fiber diet may reduce diarrhea by reducing the mechanical stimulation in the intestines, and also reduce irritation of the bowel mucosa by undigestible components.

However, some believe that a high-fiber diet may reduce symptoms by reducing watery diarrhea. This is because soluble fibers may retain water and reduce gut motility, thereby reducing the frequency of bowel movements.

A low-fiber diet is prescribed for individuals with partial obstruction due to Crohn disease, so the undigestable fiber does not become lodged in the narrowed portion of the intestine, causing a complete obstruction. Individuals with this condition should stay away from foods that cannot be fully digested such as corn, nuts, seeds, popcorn, and some vegetables used in Chinese food, including snow peas, water chestnuts, and bamboo shoots.

Nonintestinal Complications

Although Crohn disease and ulcerative colitis are inflammatory bowel diseases, they have a number of extraintestinal or systemic manifestations that are related to the autoimmune phenomenon. Some occur in individuals with either disease; some are particular to one or the other. Upwards of one-third of those with either

Crohn disease or ulcerative colitis will at some time suffer from one of these related maladies. The most frequent are arthralgia and arthritis, osteoporosis, kidney stones, gallstones, sclerosing cholangitis, fatty liver, eye inflammation, and skin inflammations.

Some of these conditions occur in conjunction with flare-ups; others precede flare-ups. In some cases, the disorders appear before any intestinal symptoms do, and are diagnostic indicators. Most of the time these conditions resolve over time and with treatment, although in rare instances they become major complications in and of themselves.

We still don't understand why these extraintestinal ailments occur, or why they occur in some people with Crohn disease or ulcerative colitis and not in others. It probably has something to do with a malfunction in the immune system, but no specific mechanism has yet been found.

Arthralgia and Arthritis

Over one quarter of those with Crohn disease or ulcerative colitis suffer from some sort of joint involvement. As a general rule, these conditions improve as the bowel symptoms dissipate, and cause no lasting damage.

Arthralgia, or aching joints, is the most common problem. Arthralgia should not be confused with arthritis, which is inflammation of the joint. Acetaminophen (the active ingredient in Tylenol and some other over-the-counter pain relievers) is usually sufficient for this discomfort.

Monoarthritis attacks one joint only, often a knee. This is the most common true arthritis that affects those with Crohn disease or ulcerative colitis. Redness and swelling (inflammation) are present.

Polyarthritis attacks several joints. It often occurs bilaterally (both knees or both wrists, for example), and it sometimes migrates from one set of joints to another.

Sacroileitis, a mild arthritis of the lower spine, is also common.

It causes soreness and stiffness, especially immediately after a person wakes.

All of these conditions often precede a flare-up of bowel symptoms by days or weeks. Medications used to reduce the intestinal inflammation also reduce these inflammations, and they usually resolve as the bowel symptoms do. (Medications will be discussed in chapter 5.)

A more disabling kind of arthritis associated with inflammatory bowel disease, which often does not resolve, is ankylosing spondylitis. This condition, which attacks the spine and sometimes the shoulders, hips, and knees, is rare. In its most severe form, the spine becomes rigid, severely limiting mobility and necessitating continued medical treatment for affected persons.

It has been noted that some individuals who take nonsteroidal anti-inflammatory drugs (NSAIDs) such as Motrin or Advil to relieve arthritis pain sometimes develop colitis, and that some people with IBD experience a worsening of their underlying condition from taking NSAIDs. It is therefore difficult for a doctor to know the best way to treat IBD patients who also have arthritis. The data is conflicting on whether NSAIDs are safe for IBD patients, but most doctors allow their patients with IBD to use NSAIDs.

However, this fact needs to be clearly noted in the patient's chart in case the regular doctor is away and the patient has to be seen urgently. In addition, the individual has to understand that the NSAIDs could potentially cause a worsening of the underlying IBD symptoms and that he or she should call the doctor immediately if symptoms worsen. In that case, taking the patient off the NSAIDs is usually the first step taken.

Osteoporosis

Osteoporosis is the loss of bone density through depletion of minerals, primarily calcium. Osteoporosis is a natural process that occurs because of aging. Most people over seventy have some reduction in bone density. One in four women have an early onset of osteoporosis after menopause. The primary symptoms are low back pain, loss of height, and fractures of the vertebrae, hips, and wrists.

Individuals who have Crohn disease or ulcerative colitis and have been treated with corticosteroids such as prednisone are at higher risk for developing osteoporosis, because the steroids damage their ability to absorb calcium. This condition is known as secondary osteoporosis. However, evidence shows that all people with Crohn disease or ulcerative colitis are at higher risk for primary osteoporosis. The reasons are not clear, but the guess is that a diet low in calcium because of lactose intolerance, as well as general malabsorption of nutrients, plays a role in the situation. The disease process itself may also be partly to blame. Some bone loss may be caused by inflammatory mediators.

All individuals with IBD, even those who have never been treated with steroids, should be screened for osteoporosis, and then treated if they have the condition. Treatments for osteoporosis seem to be as effective for those with IBD as for anyone else. With synthetic lactase, calcium-fortified foods, and calcium supplements available, it should be possible for all those with Crohn disease or ulcerative colitis to increase their calcium intake and reduce their chances of becoming debilitated by osteoporosis.

In addition, the National Osteoporosis Foundation recommends that anyone at risk for osteoporosis begin an exercise regimen to strengthen the bones in the back and hips and maintain flexibility. Those who already have signs of osteoporosis should ask their doctor whether a referral to a specialist in physical medicine is appropriate in order to create an appropriate plan.

Kidney Stones

Kidney stones occur when the kidneys do not excrete all of the oxalate in the body, and some crystallizes. Those with severe Crohn disease of the ileum and those who have had the ileum removed are most likely to produce kidney stones. Also, dehydration from severe diarrhea creates a situation favorable for formation of kidney stones.

Reducing the intake of oxalate-rich foods (spinach, beets, turnips, tea, and cola) and increasing fluid intake are the best ways to reduce the chances of developing a kidney stone.

Gallstones

Individuals with Crohn disease of the ileum are also more prone to have gallstones than is the general public. The diseased ileum does not absorb bile salts, which means that cholesterol cannot be solubilized in bile. Malabsorption of bile leads to depleted bile stores, which in turn leads to the formation of stones. A low-fat diet helps reduce the possibility of gallstones. Sometimes the gallbladder must be removed because of gallstones.

Sclerosing Cholangitis

Sclerosing cholangitis, sometimes called primary sclerosing cholangitis, is a condition in which the bile ducts both within the liver and outside it become narrowed. The condition occurs more frequently with ulcerative colitis than with Crohn disease. Symptoms are abdominal pain, fever, chills, and jaundice. Because pain, fever, and chills are symptoms of inflammatory bowel disease in general, it is important for doctors to be especially vigilant for signs of jaundice in a person with IBD. Blood tests now make it possible to diagnose the condition before it causes symptoms or problems. If untreated, sclerosing cholangitis often progresses to cirrhosis of the liver, and progressive disease can necessitate a liver transplant.

The combination of inflammatory bowel disease and sclerosing cholangitis may be a unique form of the disorder. Individuals with both conditions, especially those with ulcerative colitis, tend to have more rectal sparing disease, the presence of backwash ileitis, and generally milder disease. However, they are at higher risk for developing colon cancer, which typically is right sided.

Fatty Liver

Fatty liver is a more common complication of Crohn disease or ulcerative colitis than is sclerosing cholangitis. The liver of individuals with Crohn disease or ulcerative colitis may become infiltrated with fatty deposits. This does not come from a diet high in fat but rather from a disturbance of liver metabolism. Poor nutrition and treatment with corticosteroids has been shown to lead to this condition. It is usually mild, and resolves with improvement in the underlying bowel condition and with the end of steroid treatment. Fatty liver causes no symptoms, and is generally detected as the result of mild abnormalities in liver function tests.

Eye Inflammation

Eye inflammation characterized by redness and soreness of one eye and sensitivity to light occasionally occurs in those with Crohn disease or ulcerative colitis, usually immediately preceding a flare-up. These symptoms should receive a prompt evaluation by an ophthalmologist in order to prevent permanent eye damage.

The condition usually resolves as the bowel symptoms do. Topical steroid creams are used on the eye, and occasionally steroid injections are required.

Skin Inflammations

Those with inflammatory bowel disease are afflicted with a number of different skin inflammations. Again, these often occur immediately preceding a flare-up of bowel symptoms. Among them are the following.

Erythema nodosum, or "red bumps," are tender nodules about one-half inch in diameter that usually occur on the shins or calves. They are quite common in younger women, less common in younger men, and very rare in older individuals. This condition usually resolves as the bowel symptoms calm down.

Pyoderma, or "pus in the skin," is, thankfully, a rare condition that causes deep and chronic ulcers in the skin of the shins and ankles and occasionally the calves. Again, the condition is most common in younger women. Although most lesions heal in time after bowel symptoms have calmed, some are so deep and long-standing that skin grafts are required.

Aphthous stomatitis (sores in the mouth) are shallow ulcerations on the inside of the mouth, between the gum and lower lip or along the sides and base of the tongue. Again, they usually resolve as the bowel symptoms subside, and can be treated with topical medication.

Special Situations

Although every individual who has Crohn disease or ulcerative colitis should be considered a "special situation" and should be treated as an individual with unique needs, a few groups need some specific attention.

Children

A friend tells this story. Her sister's son, twelve years old, was diagnosed one spring with Crohn disease. He had been feeling progressively poorer through the previous fall and winter, with fevers, abdominal pains, and diarrhea. Always on the small side, the boy had been falling farther and farther behind his classmates in terms of height, weight, and development of secondary sex characteristics.

Although frightened by the diagnosis of Crohn disease, the boy's mother was relieved at least to know what the problem was after all the testing; however, she was anxious about her son going to overnight camp that summer. She called the camp director to request that her son's counselor be informed of the boy's condition, and asked if a counselor could possibly be assigned who knew something about the disease and would be sensitive to a child with some special medical needs.

No problem, the director said. All of the camp's counselors knew about inflammatory bowel disease. The camp, involved with one of the Jewish youth movements, had traditionally had a population heavily weighted toward families of Eastern European background. Over one-third of the campers, as well as the counselors and other staff, had either Crohn disease or ulcerative colitis.

This child was extremely lucky, finding himself immersed almost immediately after being diagnosed in a community that could show him in concrete terms how to have a fulfilling life despite his disease. Many other children are not as lucky. They are thrust by themselves into a frightening world of doctors, hospitals, pain, and fear.

The medical community became aware only in the last quarter of the twentieth century that Crohn disease and ulcerative colitis afflict children and young teens in large numbers. This information was now available for two reasons. One was the increasing number of diagnostic studies being done of youngsters suffering from the constellation of symptoms that adults have— chronic diarrhea, pain, bloating, nausea and vomiting, and weight loss. The other was the undertaking of retrospective studies of adults with Crohn disease or ulcerative colitis in which people were asked detailed questions about symptoms, including how long these had been present.

Nutritional deficiency is a major issue in the treatment of children and adolescents with inflammatory bowel disease. Youngsters are growing machines, and although they may not show significant weight loss, a failure to grow and a backsliding on height and weight charts should be a signal that something is amiss and needs further investigation.

For many children, taking in enough calories to fight off the bowel inflammation and extraintestinal symptoms and have normal growth at the same time is nearly impossible. Malaise, depression, and pain after eating often combine to create a lack of appetite, creating a vicious cycle.

The indications for surgery in children are essentially the same as for adults, and will be discussed in chapter 5.

People in the Childbearing Years

One of the major times for onset of Crohn disease and ulcerative colitis is from ages twenty to thirty, the prime childbearing years. Questions about fertility (both male and female) and about pregnancy are of great importance to a number of individuals who live with these diseases.

In and of themselves, neither Crohn disease nor ulcerative colitis has any effect on fertility.

In women, active disease can affect fertility. This is not so much an issue of mechanical malfunctions but rather of the underlying fever, anemia, and possible fistulas or infection. Gastroenterologists and obstetricians alike believe that, if a flare-up occurs while a woman is trying to conceive, the best idea is to focus first on beating back the disease, after which she can continue the effort.

Some medications used to treat inflammatory bowel disease, most notably sulfasalazine, decrease sperm count and sperm motility. While some couples are able to conceive while the man is taking medication, many men discontinue medication while they and their partners are engaged in this attempt.

Some of the immunoregulatory medications taken for Crohn disease or ulcerative colitis (discussed in chapter 5) may slightly increase the risk of birth defects when used by pregnant women.

If the disease is in remission at the time of conception, most pregnancies are unaffected by it. However, if the disease is active at the time of conception, it is often difficult to control during pregnancy. Many women with ulcerative colitis see a worsening of symptoms in the first trimester, while those with active Crohn disease often have their most difficult time during the third trimester. Many women also suffer flare-ups immediately postpartum. Since it is not necessary for women to discontinue medication for IBD during pregnancy, the assumption is that the change in disease process is a reaction to hormonal changes.

Women with Crohn disease and ulcerative colitis carry to full term, are able to deliver vaginally, and have healthy newborns at the same rate as women in the general population. However, women with active Crohn disease during pregnancy do have a slightly higher incidence of premature birth and stillbirth than the general population.

Surgery during pregnancy is avoided whenever possible, and only undertaken if medical management of a severe flare-up is totally unsuccessful.

Pregnant women with inflammatory bowel disease should eat the same balanced diet recommended for all pregnant women.

The Elderly

While Crohn disease and ulcerative colitis are often thought of as young people's diseases, in reality about one-fifth of new colitis cases and up to one-fourth of new Crohn cases each year are diagnosed in those over sixty. Diagnosis of late-onset inflammatory bowel disease is often difficult because the symptoms are so similar to those caused by other bowel diseases that occur more frequently in the elderly. These ailments include ischemic colitis, caused by a lack of blood flow to the bowel, irritable bowel syndrome, and diverticulosis, all of which can cause pain and diarrhea.

The incidence of colon cancer also increases with age. While many people believe the initial symptom of colon cancer is rectal bleeding, the prime symptoms of IBD (pain, fatigue, bloating, diarrhea, nausea, and low-grade fever) can also be early signs of colon cancer. It is important for the elderly not to be stoic about gastrointestinal distress but to have it checked out if it lasts more than a few days or is recurrent over a period of more than a week.

Most elderly individuals who are treated for inflammatory bowel disease, whether they are newly diagnosed or have been living with the condition for years, are able to use the same medications as younger people. However, some find that they can tolerate only low doses. In addition, since many older people have a host of medical conditions, it's important for them, their caregivers, and their physicians to coordinate closely and to watch out for reactions to combinations of medications used to treat different conditions.

Diet and nutrition can also be more complicated for the elderly. They may be limiting intake of sugar because of diabetes or salt because of high blood pressure or heart disease, and so may need a regular relationship with a nutritional counselor.

5. Treatment

Until the root causes of ulcerative colitis and Crohn disease are discovered and cures are found, these two maladies are best managed by an internist with some extra training in gastroenterology or by a gastroenterologist, if one is available.

The arsenal of medications used to treat the symptoms of Crohn disease and ulcerative colitis grows larger all the time, the result of research into the disease process and mechanisms, and of the serendipitous discovery of helpful chemical compounds. However, as yet there is no medication that can cure either condition. Although all of the mechanisms of inflammation are not understood, currently available medications seek to influence the inflammatory cascade, reversing the organic damage caused by severe and recurrent inflammation.

We continue to hope that the increased ability to treat symptoms and to curb inflammatory flare-ups early in their course will, over time, reduce the proportion of individuals with Crohn disease or ulcerative colitis who must at one time or another undergo surgery.

For ulcerative colitis, surgery, which is radical, is curative; once the diseased colon is removed there is no more colitis. But the surgical removal of the colon is also life changing, and is not a decision to be taken lightly. In the case of Crohn disease, surgery is only corrective of an immediate problem, such as obstruction, fistula, bleeding, abscess, severe perianal disease, or severe and persistent symptoms that don't respond to medical management. The disease tends to recur after surgery, sometimes quickly and sometimes many years later, usually above the place where the two portions of healthy bowel are sewn together. With either disease, surgery is sometimes necessary on an emergency basis. However, more often than not, surgery can be scheduled with some flexibility.

This chapter is divided into two sections, the first pertaining to medical management and the second to surgical interventions.

Medical Management and the Pharmaceutical Armamentarium

Medical management begins with the attempt to reduce the symptoms that cause a person to seek medical care—the initial flare-up—and to bring on a remission. After this is accomplished, the goal becomes maintenance either of total remission or of disease activity at a low enough level to permit reasonably good quality of life. Subsequent flare-ups also need to be treated medically if possible, before an individual turns to either corrective (for Crohn disease) or curative (for ulcerative colitis) surgery.

The drugs used for treatment in any one of these instances come from the same armamentarium, but are used in different doses and for different durations. In addition, the treatment patterns of doctors vary, often having to do with the custom and practice in a particular region or city and with where the doctor was trained. Finally, continued research on substances used for a number of years is leading to dose adjustments aimed at eliciting a particular response.

Data from clinical use of medications is often contradictory, with some studies showing wide variations and others showing little variation in patient outcomes between drugs or between a particular drug and a placebo. Also, combinations of drugs are often used, and it is sometimes difficult to parse the benefits of a particular one. The last large-scale, long-term studies of Crohn disease and ulcerative colitis were both carried out in the 1970s. Since then, our understanding of the disease mechanism and also the techniques in recombinant chemistry, which allow for the rapid testing of dozens of potential drugs, have led to a host of new medications for the treatment of IBD.

The situation is that medical management of individuals who

live with either of these diseases becomes more art than science, involving a basic understanding of the therapeutic benefits of each drug in combination with an intuitive sense of what benefits are actually occurring in a particular patient. This information can be derived only from close physical examination and from attentive listening and observation by the doctor over the course of a long-term doctor-patient relationship.

Some drugs work better for individuals who have ulcerative colitis and some for those with Crohn disease. In late 1998, the Food and Drug Administration approved infliximab (trade name Remicade), the first treatment exclusively for Crohn disease. The drug was approved for use by individuals with disease that does not respond to other treatments.

Four groups of drugs are generally used to treat Crohn disease and ulcerative colitis: 5-aminosalicylate compounds, corticosteroids, immunosuppressives, and antibiotics. Infliximab is a new category of treatment, a monoclonal antibody, a genetically engineered copy of an immune system protein. By the early twenty-first century, it may be possible to target the genes that create susceptibility to this disease, using a new technology called "antisense" compounds. Remicade, antisense, and other new medical avenues will be discussed in chapter 7.

5-Aminosalicylates

The active ingredient in a host of compounds used to treat inflammatory bowel disease is 5-aminosalicylic acid (5-ASA).

One compound, sulfasalazine, has been used for more than fifty years. We still do not fully understand how it works, except that it mediates the inflammatory response. Sulfasalazine produces a number of side effects that run from mild to severe, including headache, nausea, and vomiting. These side effects usually become worse as the dose is increased.

Sulfasalazine is a combination of two molecules, 5-ASA and the antibiotic sulfapyradine. It has long been known that the 5-ASA is the active ingredient, and that the sulfapyradine is what causes the side effects. Scientists spent many years researching how to deliver 5-aminosalicylic acid without attaching it to sulfapyradine, and during the 1990s non-sulfa-based 5-ASA compounds—Rowasa, Pentasa, Dipentam, and Asacol—came into general use in treating Crohn disease and ulcerative colitis.

Sulfasalazine, sold either as a generic or under the trade name Azulfidine, is more effective in treating ulcerative colitis and Crohn disease within the colon (Crohn colitis) than it is in treating Crohn disease limited to the small intestine, because the sulfapyradine is broken down in the colon by bacteria, releasing the 5-ASA into the colon.

Despite the side effects, sulfasalazine is still often the first medication used in treatment of ulcerative colitis or Crohn colitis, mostly because it is so inexpensive (the newer 5-ASA compounds are still very costly). Since the benefits are also dose dependent, an individual's response to this drug gives the doctor a good "baseline" to work from. This is a standard drug used for both maintenance and treatment of flare-ups. The standard dose is two grams (four tablets daily). The upper limit of the standard dose is four grams (eight tablets daily). High doses are six to eight grams daily. A few people tolerate doses as high as eight grams (sixteen tablets) per day. However, most people begin to suffer some side effects at four to eight tablets per day.

Many other new 5-ASA therapies were brought to market in the mid-to-late 1990s, the end product of drug development and clinical research trials that had begun a decade or more earlier. These have allowed doctors to prescribe high doses of 5-ASA for long periods of time without fear of sulfasalazine's side effects.

Also, these newer drugs allow for methods of medication administration not available with sulfasalazine for treatment of ulcerative colitis. These drugs can be administered as rectal suppositories or as enemas, as well as orally, while sulfasalazine is available only as a tablet.

For treatment of Crohn disease, some of these new medications allow 5-ASA to enter the system attached to compounds that are released in the small intestine, permitting more of the active ingredient to reach disease located there than is the case with sulfasalazine.

The active ingredient in these drugs is either mesalamine or olsalazine, each of which is a chemical compound slightly different from sulfasalazine. At present, none are available as generics. They can be found under the trade names Asacol (mcsalamine), available as a 400-milligram tablet; Pentasa (mesalamine), available as a 250-milligram capsule; Rowasa (mesalamine), available as a 500-milligram rectal suppository or a 4,000-milligram enema; and Dipentum (olsalazine), available as a 250-milligram capsule.

Evidence from clinical use throughout the 1990s has shown that all of these 5-ASA compounds are effective both in large doses as treatment for flare-ups and in lower doses as maintenance therapy for those who are in complete remission or have minor and tolerable symptoms. The maintenance dose can vary from one individual to another, and the route of administration effective for the flare-up is also the most effective route for maintenance. After surgery, those with Crohn disease are given 5-ASA medications in an effort to postpone recurrence of disease.

This clinical evidence is beginning to point to optimum doses and "correct" compounds for particular situations, although which drugs are used and in exactly what dose is still, to some degree, a matter of clinical judgment and of individual training and preference.

Despite the newer medications, sulfasalazine is the preferred first line of treatment for individuals with IBD. It is by far the most cost effective of the 5-ASA compounds. Side effects can usually be avoided by starting an individual on one pill a day and slowly increasing the dose over a period of one to two weeks. Use of the newer 5-ASA medications should be reserved for those who are allergic to sulfa-containing medications, those who prove to be intolerant to sulfasalazine, or those with small bowel disease.

Corticosteroids

Corticosteroids are powerful drugs that reduce inflammation and seem to have immunosuppressive action as well. Steroids can be administered topically by enema for ulcerative proctitis (colitis confined to the rectum) and for left-sided colitis. They can also be administered orally and, for those so sick they cannot tolerate oral feeding or for those hospitalized, intravenously or intramuscularly.

Steroids are used to treat moderate-to-severe symptoms during flare-ups. They are not effective as maintenance therapy. They are often combined with 5-ASA drugs; while 5-ASA does not enhance steroid effectiveness, steroids enhance 5-ASA effectiveness.

While steroid treatment for ulcerative colitis remains unquestioned, it is controversial for Crohn disease. Many doctors feel that the toxicity of steroids outweighs their usefulness for treating Crohn disease. However, many other doctors continue to see steroid treatment as an appropriate short-term "big gun" to beat back a severe Crohn flare-up.

Prednisone and prednisolone are the most commonly used corticosteroids for treatment of inflammatory bowel disease. These are synthetic formulations of the hormone cortisol, which is produced by the adrenal gland. Other corticosteroids used to treat either ulcerative colitis or Crohn disease include betamethasone, hydrocortisone, budesonide, and adrenocorticotropic hormone (ACTH).

Corticosteroids can produce a number of side effects, which range from annoying to dangerous. Among the annoying symptoms are a general puffiness and "mooning" of the face, acne and other skin disruptions, insomnia, tremors, night sweats, and mood disturbance. Dangerous side effects include an increase in blood pressure and severe emotional disturbances, such as psychosis and depression. Blood glucose can become elevated and potassium reduced. Long-term steroid use can lead to cataracts or glaucoma. Some individuals who are on steroid therapy also suffer from osteoporosis, a loss of bone mass. Although this is often thought of as a long-term effect, it can occur in those who take steroids for even a few months. A rare disorder called aseptic necrosis of the hip, sometimes referred to as avascular necrosis of the femoral head, can also occur.

In addition, while steroid treatment helps improve appetite in those who may have experienced severe weight loss and even malnutrition during their flare-up, continued use of the drugs means an ongoing increase in appetite and can lead to enormous weight gain, which has its own dangers.

For those with severe disease coupled with rapid weight loss and malnutrition, treatment with intravenous steroids during a period of hospitalization, together with intravenous hydration and possibly total parenteral nutrition (TPN), is often necessary.

Because steroids are such powerful drugs, and because many individuals have a certain level of anxiety—or even fear—about having to use them, it's worthwhile to take a little extra time to analyze the clinical decision making that goes into a doctor's prescribing them.

Doctors try to stick to four general rules in using steroids: (1) avoid them unless necessary; (2) use the most direct route of administration; (3) use the lowest effective dose, and taper the medication as rapidly as possible; (4) stop steroid medication before stopping other medications.

Basically, the doctor considers four questions.

Are Steroids Necessary?

Steroids are typically reserved for severe flare-ups of either Crohn disease or ulcerative colitis or for more chronic disabling symptoms that are not responsive to other medications. While people with mild-to-moderate symptoms are usually treated with 5-ASA medications, because steroids are more effective and act more rapidly they are often used in an effort to get the upper hand against a flare-up.

Some doctors use one of the numerous scoring methods for disease severity in their decision to use steroids. Others use less formal methods, taking into consideration the constellation of symptoms: pain, number of bowel movements per day, gross bleeding, fever, and weight loss.

What Route of Administration Should Be Used?

For those with limited ulcerative colitis (ulcerative proctitis or proctosigmoiditis), a directed treatment is often sufficient. People with proctitis may respond to a topical steroid foam applied via the anus. Those who have proctosigmoiditis may respond to a steroid enema.

For individuals with more extensive involvement of the colon or with Crohn disease and who are suffering a severe flare-up but who are not sick enough to require hospitalization, prednisone is given orally, in pill form. When an individual is sick enough to require hospitalization, the medication is given intravenously to ensure maximum absorption and achieve the best results.

What Should the Dose Be?

Locally administered steroid preparations come in single-dose applicator packaging. The typical dose of oral prednisone for a flare-up is forty to sixty milligrams. A typical dose for a hospitalized individual is three hundred milligrams of hydrocortisone given intravenously. These doses are tapered over a period of time, balancing the quickest possible decrease with maintenance of remission.

Doctors differ in their approach regarding the situation of an individual who has a flare-up while currently on prednisone and is tapering the dose or of someone who has recently completed a course of steroid treatment and has a flare-up. In these cases, some doctors restart the steroids at the lowest effective dose—ten to twenty milligrams—and attempt to control the symptoms while avoiding the worst side effects of steroids. Others consider this to be taking half measures and immediately go back to forty milligrams.

There is also some debate about how rapidly to taper the medication in these circumstances. Some doctors go for a rapid taper, while others use the standard reduction of five milligrams per week until the individual is at ten to twenty milligrams, then reduce more slowly and/or by smaller increments. The more rapid taper decreases the time a patient is being treated with a highly toxic substance. The slower taper is thought to give the body's adrenal system a better chance of adjusting and producing the proper amount of natural hormones.

How Should Other Medications Be Used in Conjunction with Steroids?

This question actually involves two kinds of situations. One has to do with an individual who is having an initial flare-up, or has been totally off medication for a time; the question here is how and when to add other medications. The other situation concerns an individual who has been taking either 5-ASA medications or immunomodulators (discussed in detail below) and has a flare-up; in this case the question is whether to discontinue the other medications during steroid treatment.

The answer to this two-part question really hinges on individual practice protocol. There is little research to guide doctors in how they add or subtract medications. Since individuals respond differently to each medication used, doctors usually like to add new substances slowly, to tease apart the effects and side effects of each.

A Final Caution

The bottom line regarding steroids is that, while they work wonders for many people, because of their toxicity they cannot be allowed to become a way of life for anyone. Chronic steroid use is dangerous and should be avoided at all costs.

The newer group of immunosuppressives/immunomodulators, discussed below, offers an opportunity for many patients to get off steroids. For those who do not tolerate these drugs, a longer course of steroid therapy may be necessary and useful.

But once the usefulness of steroids is in question—when they are not creating a lasting remission—other measures must be taken.

Immunosuppressives/Immunomodulators

Immunosuppressive drugs are powerful compounds that override the body's natural immune defenses. They are most widely known for their use in organ transplants to reduce the possibility of rejection of the donated organ by the host body. However, since the early 1960s, gastroenterologists have experimented with immunosuppressives in an effort to "turn off" the inappropriate inflammatory response in the bowel.

This experimentation grew from the reasoning of Swedish scientists, who reported in 1959 that antibodies to colon tissue were circulating in the blood of patients with ulcerative colitis. They reasoned that ulcerative colitis and the related Crohn disease were "autoimmune" diseases, in which the body's immune system attacks its own organs, mistaking them for invading organisms. The Swedish doctors theorized that these diseases could be treated with antimetabolite drugs, variants of the building blocks of antibody-producing cell nuclei that were used in an effort to kill these cells.

In 1962 an Australian doctor treated one patient who had ulcerative colitis with the antimetabolite 6-mercaptopurine (6-MP). The patient experienced dramatic remission that lasted for over two years of treatment with the drug and for a period after the end of treatment. Throughout the 1960s, doctors in Australia, Europe, and the United States treated patients with either 6-MP or its close relative azathioprine. They published their case reports, and in the 1970s researchers who ran the National Cooperative Crohn Disease Study (NCCDS) tested both substances against placebo.

The NCCDS results were unimpressive; few patients did better on the drugs than on placebo. However, it is now known, after twenty years of empirical use and further careful study, that neither the Australian doctors nor those who conducted the tests as part of the NCCDS gave the treatment long enough for it to become effective. (It is important to understand that, while none of these drugs has Food and Drug Administration approval for use in IBD, since they are approved for use in organ transplants, doctors can prescribe them "off label" for any condition.)

Both 6-MP (trade name Purinethol) and azathioprine (trade name Imuran) inhibit T-helper lymphocyte cells, which play a large role in the inflammatory process.

Doctors continue to refine the dosing of these medications, so that today they are considered immunoregulators rather than immunosuppressives. They are used more often in Crohn disease than in ulcerative colitis. In the 1980s most doctors limited use of these medications to those with severe disease unresponsive to conventional treatmen and to those with long-term steroid dependence. Today, the drugs are often used early in the treatment of a severe flare-up, either in conjunction with the 5-ASA compounds or after a short course of steroids. They are also used to treat fistulas, and even as maintenance therapy.

It often takes three to six months for the benefits of immunoregulators to begin appearing. Individuals taking them are required to have regular blood tests to make sure that a steep reduction in white blood cells does not occur, which would create a risk for severe infection. Fewer than 10 percent of individuals cannot tolerate these medications; such people can develop fever and rash, nausea and vomiting, hepatitis or pancreatitis.

Experiments have been conducted with cyclosporin, a powerful immunosuppressive, in refractory Crohn disease and ulcerative colitis and in severe attacks that do not respond to high doses of steroids. Short-term results were good in the group of ulcerative colitis patients unresponsive to intravenous steroids during hospitalization. Recent evidence shows that a remission induced by intravenous cyclosporin can be maintained by long-term use of 6-MP.

Some scientists are working on a way to track clinical response to 6-MP treatment through a blood metabolite. If the metabolite level is kept in an appropriate range, patients may respond better to the treatment.

Methotrexate, an immunoregulator used in treating rheumatoid arthritis and psoriasis, has also been used experimentally in both ulcerative colitis and Crohn disease. Although there is no conclusive evidence via double-blind studies of its effectiveness, it has proved effective in individual cases, and is used with patients who don't respond to other immunoregulators or who suffer side effects.

Antibiotics

Evidence is pointing increasingly to bacteria as an important element in Crohn disease. Research is being conducted into finding bacterial agent(s) that trigger the inflammatory response. In addition, for those with Crohn disease of the terminal ileum and damage to the ileocecal valve, bacteria from the colon commonly back up into the ileum. This causes a condition known as bacterial overgrowth, in which bacteria flourish in the small intestine, where they are not normally present. Bacterial overgrowth causes problems with nutrient absorption, as well as bloating, gas, and diarrhea.

For this reason antibiotic treatment is increasingly common in Crohn disease. Broad-spectrum antibiotics such as ciprofloxacin (Cipro), clarithromycin (Biaxin), and Ampicillin are often used in a short course of treatment in an effort to reduce the bacterial overgrowth and calm the infection. Scientists have recently attached Cipro to a budesonide-controlled capsule that releases the medication in the ileum.

The most commonly used antibiotic is metronidazole (Flagyl), which is usually given in a four-to-eight-week course of treatment during flare-ups. The drug often induces remission, but does not maintain it. Flagyl also helps heal fistulas. Side effects are more annoying than dangerous, and include metallic taste, loss of appetite, yeast infections, and numbness of the hands and feet. Anyone taking Flagyl should be careful about alcohol consumption; in some people even a sip of wine or beer causes vomiting.

A cousin of metronidazole, another nitroimidazole antibiotic called omidazole, has also been tested and has shown some effectivenss.

Surgical Treatments

Indications for Surgery in Ulcerative Colitis

Surgery for ulcerative colitis involves removal of the colon. This is a curative procedure, since ulcerative colitis is confined to the colon, and, once the colon has been removed, the disease does not reappear in the small intestine above the suture line.

Surgery can be done on an elective, an urgent, or an emergency basis. Emergency surgery must be performed immediately; urgent surgery is usually performed within days, and the individual remains hospitalized until the surgery; elective surgery can be scheduled at the convenience of the individual (within reason).

Emergency surgery is necessary for three different conditions: perforation, severe bleeding, and toxic megacolon. All of these conditions are uncommon.

If an ulceration perforates the wall of the colon, bowel contents and air enter the abdominal cavity, which causes peritonitis, a dangerous infection.

Bleeding occurs frequently in ulcerative colitis, and even severe bleeding can usually be treated in the hospital, with intravenous steroids and transfusion. Occasionally bleeding is so sudden, and so massive, that emergency surgery becomes necessary.

In toxic megacolon, the colon loses its muscle tone, fills with air and fecal material, and distends. It usually occurs in individuals who are already quite ill. Sometimes toxic megacolon can be treated medically with high-dose steroids and antibiotics and decompression of the colon using nasogastric and rectal tubes. If the situation doesn't resolve in a matter of hours, emergency surgery is performed. If it does resolve, surgery is usually still necessary because of the likelihood of recurrence of toxic megacolon, but the procedure can be delayed for days or weeks so the individual can gain strength.

Urgent surgery is carried out in the case of fulminant colitis, which can lead to toxic megacolon if it does not resolve or is not dealt with surgically. Fulminant colitis is severe diarrhea, accompanied by bleeding and fever, that lasts for many hours. Again, sometimes this condition responds to treatment with high-dose intravenous steroids and antibiotics in a hospital setting. Some doctors try cyclosporin as well. Oral feedings are stopped. If the situation doesn't resolve in about a week, surgery is performed.

When emergency or urgent surgery is necessary for individuals with ulcerative colitis, a subtotal colectomy is usually performed; the colon is removed but the rectum left in place, and a standard ileostomy is constructed. An ostomy is a surgically constructed opening in the abdomen from which the intestine protrudes so that bowel contents can be eliminated. If it is appropriate for the individual, the small intestine can be connected to the rectum at a later date, or the rectum can be removed.

Elective surgery for ulcerative colitis is an option for individuals who have long-standing disease with constant flare-ups, so that their quality of life is severely impaired. Although many people consider the colectomy surgery an admission of failure and fear the unknown of postsurgical life, the overwhelming majority comment that they should have had the procedure done earlier because of the radical improvement in their quality of life.

Another reason for elective colectomy in those with ulcerative colitis is the presence of colon cancer or precancerous cellular changes known as dysplasia. There is an increased risk of colon cancer in individuals with an eight-year or longer history of ulcerative colitis; the incidence increases for those whose entire colon is involved.

Surgical Options for Ulcerative Colitis

For many years, proctocolectomy (removal of the entire colon and rectum) and ileostomy was the only surgical option for those in need of surgery for ulcerative colitis. Indeed, even after new surgical techniques appeared in the 1970s, the total colectomy and traditional ileostomy continued to be the "gold standard" (fig. 5.1).

A variation of this surgery is the construction of a so-called continent ileostomy. Instead of the ileostomy constantly draining bowel contents into an external bag fitted to the side of the abdomen, the ileostomy is constructed with a nipple valve, and bowel contents are eliminated regularly during the day through a short, rigid catheter inserted through the valve. An internal pouch for collecting and holding the waste is created from the small-intestine tissue and stitched to the inside of the abdomen.

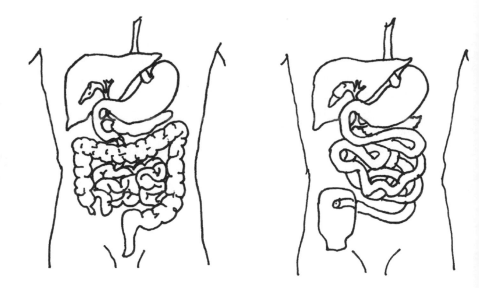

FIG. 5.1 Left: Normal gastrointestinal tract. Right: Gastrointestinal tract after total colectomy and external ostomy.

Today, however, more people are opting for a surgical procedure that allows for a more natural elimination of waste. This is done with an ileal pouch-anal anastomosis, commonly referred to as a J-pouch (fig. 5.2).

This procedure is possible because ulcerative colitis is a disease that only affects the inner lining, or mucosa, of the colon and rectum. The colon is removed. The inner lining of the rectum is stripped off the outer muscle walls, and the anus and anal sphincter are left intact. The ileum, the end of the small intestine, is brought down to the rectum. An internal pouch in the shape of a "J" is created from the ileal tissue (sometimes

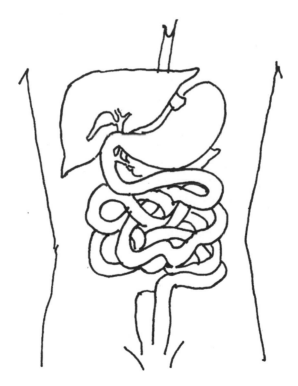

FIG. 5.2 Gastrointestinal tract after total colectomy and ileal pouch, anal anastomosis.

referred to as a neorectum). A temporary ostomy is created for six to eight weeks until the new pouch and rectum heal. A newer surgical technique sometimes used includes a stapling device and a small cuff of rectal mucosa that is left behind.

Most people who have this procedure report relatively normal bowel function, with six to eight soft bowel movements a day. Thirty to 40 percent of people who have the surgery will at some time experience a condition known as "pouchitis," a nonspecific inflammation of the J-pouch. They may experience fever, diarrhea, fatigue, anemia, weight loss, and even joint pain. Pouchitis usually responds to a short course of treatment with antibiotics, and can also be treated with the 5-ASA compound Rowesa administered as a suppository or enema. A serological test called an ANCA test may help predict incipient pouchitis.

Fewer than 10 percent of J-pouch surgeries fail to perform satisfactorily. If they do, they can be converted to either a standard or a continent ostomy. It's important to remember, however, that pouchitis also occurs in continent ileostomies.

Indications for Surgery for Crohn Disease

As with ulcerative colitis, surgery for Crohn disease sometimes must be undertaken in an emergency, but more often is classified as urgent or even elective. Unlike surgery for ulcerative colitis, however, surgery for Crohn disease is not curative; it is only corrective of an immediate complication. Between two-thirds and three-quarters of individuals who suffer from Crohn disease will undergo surgery at some point.

Reasons for emergency surgery are perforation, toxic megacolon, bleeding, and sudden total obstruction. Urgent surgery is performed for subtotal obstruction, for fistulas or abscesses that do not respond quickly to medical treatment, and when cancer is diagnosed. Elective surgery is undertaken for chronic partial obstruction or persistent fistulas, or when medical management fails to control symptoms and quality of life is severely impaired.

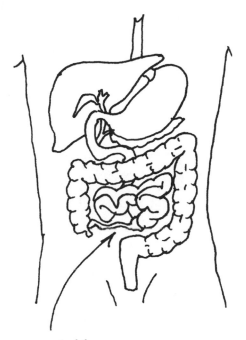

FIG. 5.3 Stricture at terminal ileum.

The most common surgery for individuals with Crohn disease is partial intestinal resection with reanastomosis (reconnection). This is performed to remove areas of the bowel significantly damaged by disease and can be done anywhere in the small or large intestine. Figure 5.3 shows a narrowing, called a stricture, at the terminal ileum, and figure 5.4 shows a partial resection with reanastomosis to remove the severely narrowed terminal ileum, as well as the ileocecal valve, appendix, and the cecum.

This surgery is performed to remove either a partial or total obstruction. Surgery to correct obstruction is straightforward. The diseased bowel is removed and two ends of healthy bowel sewn together. The goal of removing as much diseased tissue as possible is weighed against that of preserving as much intestine as possible. A temporary ostomy is sometimes required to allow for healing.

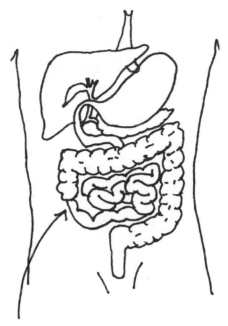

FIG. 5.4 Resection of stricture and small portion of colon (ileocolectomy) with anastomosis.

Crohn disease frequently recurs above the site of the original resection, often immediately above. There is about a 20 percent recurrence of self-reported symptoms at two years, 30 percent at three years, and 50 percent at five years. Most of these recurrences can be treated medically, but estimates are that up to 50 percent of people will have to have a second resection, and as many as 25 percent will have to have three or more resections. Beginning an individual on medication immediately after surgery has become more standard practice since the mid 1990s, and the hope is that this will cut down on the recurrence of clinical symptoms and the need for successive resections.

In addition, some individuals who have had a resection will need surgery at another time to drain an abscess or close a fistula.

These statistics show why it is so important to preserve as much intestine as possible in each surgery. At some point, so much small intestine can be resected that an individual can end up with "short gut syndrome," in which he or she is unable to maintain nutritional needs through oral feedings, and must rely on total parenteral nutrition (TPN). Fortunately, this is extremely rare.

Small areas of obstruction can often be treated with a technique called strictureplasty, in which the narrowed area is cut lengthwise, then sewn across in an effort to widen the narrowing (fig. 5.5). The procedure has been used just since the 1980s; before that, surgeons felt that the only way to deal with diseased tissue was to remove it. Today the procedure is done frequently, and it is not uncommon for a surgeon performing a resection of a significant area also to perform

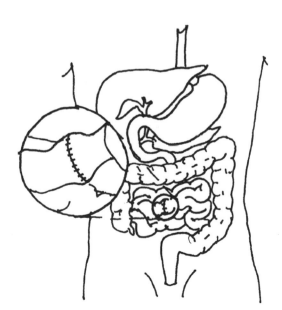

FIG. 5.5 Correction of small stricture by strictureplasty.

numerous strictureplasties to open other areas that might become troublesome over time.

Surgical procedures to correct fistulas that connect the intestine to other intestinal loops or to internal organs are also relatively straightforward; in these cases surgery is an adjunct to continued medical therapy. Surgery to correct anorectal fistulas, fissures, or abscesses and ano- or rectovaginal fistulas is far more delicate and complex, and often requires the assistance of a urologist or gynecologist.

6. The Mind/Body Connection

It is almost shocking today to read medical literature from the first half of this century, when doctors were starting to put names to the confluence of symptoms we now know as Crohn disease and ulcerative colitis. At one time the "ulcerative colitis personality" was seriously discussed, and even now some people retain the misperception that these disorders are psychosomatic, brought on by underlying psychological problems.

Today, we are only at the beginning of a true understanding of mind-body interactions and how they affect diseases. We now know that individuals can't "give" themselves ulcerative colitis or Crohn disease. But we also know that the way an individual responds psychologically and emotionally to IBD—or to any chronic illness, for that matter—can have an effect on treatment and on quality of life. We know, too, that stress does have an effect on the body, making it more difficult for the immune system to do its work.

Chronic Illness

It can be said that living with a chronic illness is like having a second full-time job. It is a constant struggle of management: management of medication, of appointments with health care providers, and of one's own inner resources.

Individuals who have Crohn disease or ulcerative colitis must constantly marshal their strength. If you are such a person, while it is not necessary to "baby" yourself, it is important to carry out the regimens of daily living that in the past have helped you to maintain maximum health. These include (1) sticking to the diet that works for you; (2) getting enough sleep, even if you are feeling well and even if that sometimes means saying no to work, community, social, or even family events that require late nights; (3) taking prescribed medication, even if you are feeling well (maintenance doses are meant to do just that—maintain well-being); (4) keeping regularly scheduled appointments with your gastroenterologist or internist and any other medical practitioners who are monitoring your condition, even if you are feeling well.

Over the course of a lifetime with an illness, an individual will almost certainly experience personal feelings resembling those of people who are grieving, or who have been traumatized, or who have a terminal illness—anger, disbelief, fear, denial, bargaining, resignation, and depression. It's important to recognize these feelings in yourself or in the one you love or help to care for. Realize that for most, each of these feelings will be transient, and a support system of family, friends, colleagues or classmates, community or congregation acquaintances, and support groups of those similarly affected will help them through the difficult times.

But for those who have been ill for a long time, or who are in a period when their disease is debilitating, the normal support system may not provide sufficient help. There is a time and a place for professional counseling, and a number of social workers, psychologists, and psychiatrists are making a specialty of patients who suffer from chronic illness.

Effects on Family

Having a chronically ill family member is stressful for every person in the household. At the same time, the family is the central unit in the support system for any person who suffers from Crohn disease, ulcerative colitis, or any other chronic illness.

If the affected individual is a child, the adults' lives are turned upside down, and siblings often feel a lack of love and attention as their parents' efforts are largely directed toward the ill child.

If the ill individual is a parent, a disproportionate burden of family life can fall on the healthy spouse, turning that person into a de facto single parent. Children can feel uneasy about having a parent who is unable to participate in their lives, who is frequently in the hospital or at home in bed and thus cannot attend school, music, athletic, or other events.

Side effects from medication are another complication. In addition to suffering from the chronic fatigue involved with a flare-up, some people experience headache or nausea from medications. Steroid use frequently leads to mood changes and depression.

Regardless of which family member is ill, Crohn disease or ulcerative colitis is debilitating for the entire family. Flare-ups often occur suddenly, causing plans to be changed. Outings may need to be planned around proximity to toilet facilities. Travel is sometimes difficult, as changes in water and food, as well as sleep disturbances caused by jet lag, can cause drastic changes in bowel habits.

Hospitalizations

Hospitals are not restful places. The movement in medicine to get patients out of the hospital as quickly as possible, evident since the 1980s, is not only an issue of reducing medical costs. People's overall mental and physical well-being is enhanced if they can spend more time recuperating at home in a normal setting and getting the treatments they need on an outpatient or even a home-health basis. Despite this, many, if not most, individuals who suffer from Crohn disease or ulcerative colitis will be hospitalized at least once because of the disease. These hospitalizations will be either to the surgical or to the general medical service, except in extreme cases, where intensive care will be required.

Between one-third and three-quarters of those with Crohn disease will require surgery at least once to correct or repair a stricture (narrowing of a portion of the intestine), a complete or nearly complete obstruction, a fistula, or an abscess. A number of those with colitis will ultimately seek a surgical cure. Many others will spend time in the hospital for medical treatment of complications, including the beginning of TPN treatments.

Hospital stays are stressful not only for the person in treatment but for the entire family. The patient feels the stress of doing battle with the disease to the exclusion of other activities, and has the sense that in some way the disease has "won" by forcing a hospitalization. For other family members, the stress comes from having the routines of family life broken.

However, the hospital experience can be used as an opportunity to regroup, to regain strength and a feeling of general well-being; it can almost be considered a "forced vacation." It's important to remember what was said earlier: that dealing with a chronic illness is like having a second full-time job, or a third if you are working and raising a family. Catching up on reading or writing letters is a more useful way to spend hospital time than trying to do office work. Some people find keeping a journal of their thoughts and feelings helpful.

If the hospitalization is due to a planned surgery, proper "training" may shorten the stay and speed your recovery. A high-protein diet and the most physical conditioning possible—bike riding, walking, or using a treadmill—can get you up and around the corridors soon after surgery. If the hospitalization is unplanned, it is harder to control the situation.

Remember, in the hospital you are under the care of the hospital staff as well as of your own private doctor. You need to talk to everyone, and questioning why someone wants to do something is not wrong. If you feel uncomfortable with any procedure that you are asked to undergo by the resident medical staff, ask to have it confirmed by your own doctor.

You are entitled to know about all of the medications that are being administered and to understand the results of any diagnostic or lab procedures. Again, if you feel that the hospital staff is not responding appropriately to your questions, ask to speak to your own doctor.

You have the right to be visited by clergy of your choice and also not to be visited by hospital chaplains if that is your wish. You can make this known at the time of your admission.

Individuals have different desires regarding hospital visits. Some want the constant stimulation of family and friends; others would rather be left more or less on their own. No one wants to have the visitors' chairs occupied by those who are anxious or angry. You're the patient; if your family or friends have difficulty being with you and responding to your situation, it's all right to tell them that you'll see them when you get home.

Body Image

Although there are typically few, if any, outward signs that an individual has Crohn disease or ulcerative colitis, feelings about body image constitute an important psychological component of IBD. A person may worry constantly about disrupting the social or business flow of the day because of the need to use the toilet many times and may fear losing bowel control and soiling clothes. Steroids can have outward physical effects, such as facial "mooning," an increase in facial hair, and skin blemishes. And those who have had an ostomy may wear apparatus, albeit under clothing.

Body image is a special issue for adolescents with Crohn disease or ulcerative colitis. Many have some degree of retardation in growth and sexual maturation, this occurring at a time of heightened awareness regarding their own physical characteristics and concerns about whether they are perceived as "attractive."

Fear of Colo-Rectal Cancer

Because those with Crohn disease and ulcerative colitis have an increased rate of colo-rectal cancer, affected individuals may develop a major fear of that disease. The increase in incidence is far more for those with colitis, especially if the entire colon is involved (pancolitis). While the risk is dependent on the amount of colon involved, it is not dependent on the severity of the inflammation.

The recommendation is that those with colitis begin to have regularly scheduled screening colonoscopies beginning eight years after diagnosis and those with Crohn disease fifteen years after diagnosis. People with Crohn disease who have significant disease in the colon are often screened beginning eight years after diagnosis, as if they had colitis.

Researchers are making an effort both to find the link between inflammatory bowel disease and colo-rectal cancer and to determine how best to treat those with IBD who show possible precancerous tissue changes. Scientists from the United Kingdom have recently suggested that the risk of IBD sufferers developing colon cancer may not be as great as previously thought. However, scientists at two medical centers in the United States caution that it is important to treat low-grade dysplasia, because it can very quickly advance to high-grade dysplasia, a dangerous precancerous condition.

Finally, scientists and doctors are creating better strategies for dealing with IBD patients who have polyps. The question is whether polyps should be seen to represent evidence of dysplasia, or whether they should be seen as random, as in an individual without IBD. In general, the thought is that if the polyp occurs in a segment of normal bowel, it should be seen simply as a polyp. But when it occurs in the setting of colitis, it should be examined more closely and rechecked more frequently.

A Necessary Strategy

Because Crohn disease and ulcerative colitis are chronic conditions, it is important to create a long-term strategy for managing the diseases. Such a program includes developing strong relationships with professionals, especially a gastroenterologist you feel comfortable with. Other specialists who may be necessary parts of the team are a nutritionist, a surgeon, and a psychological counselor.

It is also a good idea to have a strong nonprofessional support group of family, friends, and others who understand your situation and empathize with you as you pass through the inevitable difficult periods. Finally, remaining informed of the latest research into causes and treatments is important. This can be done through peers and/or use of various resources such as those listed in the appendices of this book.

Mind/Body Medicine and IBD

Mind/body therapies can be quite useful; they can help individuals with Crohn disease or ulcerative colitis manage pain, can contribute to a sense of well-being, and can give sufferers some feeling of control in a situation where, in medical terms, they have little or none. While there is no proof that these therapies can undo the cellular damage done by inflammatory bowel disease, much anecdotal evidence suggests that such techniques can provide great relief for many with IBD.

Many people argue that these results are due simply to a "placebo effect"—the sense that something is being done although nothing really is. But others argue that the effects on subjective symptoms such as pain, fatigue, and nausea are real, even if there is no change in the disease process itself or in the objective signs.

We believe that, as long as mind/body therapies are used in an adjunctive way and not as a substitute for Western scientific medicine, they can be useful. Those who live with IBD and seek complementary therapies should try to establish relationships with practitioners who agree that their methods are an attempt to alleviate discomfort and do not claim the possibility of a cure.

What do we mean by mind/body therapies? They are therapies designed to help patients relax and to, in effect, disentangle their consciousness from their pain and discomfort. Mind/body therapies are one of six categories of "alternative" treatments that the National Institute of Health's Office of Alternative Medicine (NIH-OAM) has been studying for nearly a decade.

During the 1990s, alternative medicine was discovered by scientific practitioners, and health care scholars began studying how Americans integrated alternative therapies with Western therapies in their approach to health care. In 1993, *The New England Journal of Medicine* published a study showing that 34 percent of all Americans had used alternative therapies in the previous year. Almost 90 percent of them had "self-referred," and only a third had informed their doctor that they were seeking alternative care.

The NIH-OAM has defined six categories of alternative medical therapies, and continues to fund researchers who are studying the sociological aspects of these kinds of therapies as well as more rigorous scientific investigators who are asking if the methods are, indeed, effective. These researchers are using traditional scientific means of experimentation, trying to produce results that can be replicated in different populations.

The six NIH-OAM categories are:

1. Diet, nutrition, and lifestyle. This category includes the practice of macrobiotics, use of megavitamins, adherence to specialized diets, and general lifestyle changes, as well as the addition of supplements such as fish oil. Many argue that diet, nutrition, and lifestyle changes are hardly "alternative," having become part of the standard regimen prescribed by many primary care doctors. Certainly, most gastroenterologists believe that finding the proper diet, maintaining good nutrition, and creating a lifestyle that allows an individual with IBD to maintain the best health while participating in as many family, work, and social activities as possible is important. They are usually willing to refer their patients to nutritionists and to allow patients to engage in specialized diets, as long as the individuals agree to be monitored regularly for nutritional deficiency.

2. Mind/body medicine. Included here are biofeedback, guided imagery, hypnotherapy, sound/music therapy, relaxation techniques, and even prayer.

3. Ethnotherapies. Such therapies include acupuncture, traditional Asian herbal compounds, homeopathy and naturopathy; Hispanic, African, Afro-American, and Afro-Caribbean healing techniques; Ayurvedic medicine; and American Indian healing techniques.

Traditional Chinese herbal compounds are generally frowned upon for treatment of IBD, as are naturopathic or homeopathic remedies. "Intestinal" herbal remedies were generally created to deal with parasitic or bacterial illnesses. There is no evidence that Chinese herbal compounds have any effect on IBD, and they may, in fact, produce adverse results when combined with standard medical therapies such as 5-ASA compounds, steroids, or immunoregulators.

Homeopathy and naturopathy are problematic. Homeopathy works on the principle that "like cures like." Homeopathic "cures" are minute dilutions of plant, animal, or mineral matter thought to be disease-causing agents. Naturopathy seeks natural cures to illness through the use of standard medical tests, nutritional and herbal supplements, and elimination diets. Neither of these practices seems to work for people with inflammatory bowel disease, although some people with IBD do seek treatment from such practitioners. Most gastroenterologists will not treat patients if they are also being seen by a naturopath or a homeopath, although some will work in conjunction with these practitioners.

Acupuncture has shown some promise in relieving anxiety and pain, thereby aiding patients' subjective feelings of well-being.

4. Structural and energy techniques. These include acupressure, chiropractic, reflexology, Rolfing, therapeutic massage, and therapeutic touch. Again, there is no evidence that these techniques in any way change the IBD disease process. Chiropractors especially are sometimes willing to claim that their treatments can "cure" IBD; no evidence for this exists.

These techniques may assist with relaxation and relief of pain and anxiety. But they should never be used instead of care from an internist or gastroenterologist.

5. Alternative pharmaceutical and biological therapies such as antioxidants, chelation, and metabolic therapy. It cannot be demonstrated that these techniques help those with IBD in any way.

6. Bioelectric appliances. Although one study in 1998 reported that magnets relieved chronic pain, there is no evidence that bioelectric appliances can do anything to cause a change in underlying disease process.

Clearly, medical practitioners in the United States are increasingly coming to realize, if not to accept, that a number of their patients are seeking treatments from traditions other than that of Western scientific medicine. It is extremely important, however, that any alternative treatment be undertaken in a fashion complementary to medical treatment and not used as a true alternative. Such treatment should also be undertaken with the knowledge—and, we hope, the consent, after thorough discussion—of the gastroenterologist or internist who is the primary provider of care. Seeking treatment from providers who are working at cross purposes can be dangerous.

Mind/Body Treatments

We believe that mind/body treatments such as hypnosis, biofeedback, and relaxation techniques including autogenic training, progressive muscle relaxation, and meditation can help to improve quality of life for those who live with IBD. Such treatments provide people with a sense that they can put themselves in control of their pain and anxiety.

Other ways in which people may be able to control pain and anxiety are through massage, including lymphatic massage, neuromuscular massage, and Rolfing; postural therapies, including the Alexander technique, the Feldenkrais method, and the Trager method (all designed to help actors and dancers more consciously control their bodies' movements); and chiropractic or osteopathic manipulation.

Acupuncture and acupressure, both from the traditional Chinese medical repertoire, have also been shown to be effective in pain and anxiety management, and thus may provide relief for those with IBD, although no studies have been undertaken of these techniques on a population of individuals living with IBD.

None of these noninvasive techniques can harm an individual; none can have any adverse affects on medication. Therefore, although most gastroenterologists remain skeptical of their effectiveness, most will say to their patients, in effect: "If that's the way you want to spend your money, I hope you get some relief."

Prayer

Although prayer is not technically a part of mind/body medicine, it is a powerful tool in the comforting of anyone suffering from medical affliction, and may indeed provoke a positive physiological response. Surveys of Americans consistently find that between 80 and 90 percent of adults believe in a universal organizing principle of life, and most are willing to call that principle God.

The National Institute of Health Research has studied spirituality and health since the early 1990s, and has discovered that patients with chronic illnesses who use spiritual practices as adjuncts to medical care generally report benefits from these practices. In fact, there is some evidence from a Duke University study of patients undergoing coronary angioplasty that those who are being prayed for by others have better outcomes than those for whom no prayers are being offered.

Although the medical community remains mostly skeptical about the power of prayer to cure illness, or even to affect outcomes, doctors are increasingly working with spiritual leaders from a number of faiths, as well as hospital chaplains, to help chronically ill patients accept—and to help themselves accept—that while there may not always be a cure, there is always the potential for spiritual healing. As of the turn of the century, over twenty medical schools are offering classes about spirituality and its relation to patients' well-being; some schools are even considering making such classes mandatory in the near future.

The sense of spiritual healing can greatly reduce the fear, anxiety, and depression that often accompany a chronic illness such as Crohn disease or ulcerative colitis, and can thus enhance the quality of life for an individual who lives with these conditions.

7. The Search for a Cure

Clinical manifestations of inflammatory bowel disease follow a complex series of cellular changes. A number of different disease components affect these changes. We do not know to what extent each of these components influences the course of inflammatory bowel disease, whether interrupting one or more of them can break the chain, or if all must be mediated to change the course of the disease.

These components are: genetic susceptibility; an environmental factor that acts as a "priming event," possibly an early childhood illness; an imbalance in the immunoregulatory system; a second environmental factor that acts as a "triggering event," possibly a viral, bacterial, or even parasitic infection; and a state of increased permeability of the intestinal wall, sometimes referred to as a "leaky gut" (fig. 7.1).

Current research focuses on each of these components, as well as on issues of increasing the effectiveness of medications in current use and the development of new medications. Research is being conducted in the areas of genetics, possible infectious causes of IBD, and the inappropriate immune activity that occurs in IBD. Many researchers who focus on IBD are also

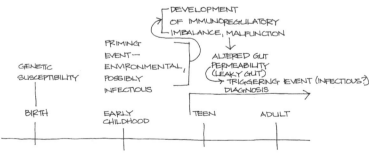

FIG. 7.1 Theoretical event timeline for onset of inflammatory bowel disease.

helped in their thinking by research that is being done on other autoimmune diseases involving the inflammatory response, such as rheumatoid arthritis, multiple sclerosis, and lupus. Basic research on the inflammatory response is helping researchers who study all of these clinical manifestations.

Genetics

To date, no gene has been identified that alone is sufficient for the development of either Crohn disease or ulcerative colitis. Currently, most genetic research is focused on chromosomes 12 and 16, although there is some research being done on chromosome 1p, 3, 4 and 6 as well. The research methodology is one that looks for genetic marker variations on these genes that show up in pairs of relatives—siblings or cousins—who have IBD more often than would be expected by chance.

Recent research at Johns Hopkins University and the University of Chicago has identified families with abnormalities on chromosomes 1p, 3q, 4q and 16. Researchers in Toronto have demonstrated a link between Crohn disease and a major histocompatibility complex on chromosome 6. Histocompatibility is the compatibility between a tissue donor and a recipient. An abnormality in histocompatibility could be what causes the autoimmune effect, in which an individual's immune system believes that his or her own tissue is a foreign body. This might be why immunoregulatory drugs given to organ recipients work in Crohn disease as well.

Other abnormalities have recently been described in genes that help control the body's response to inflammation. These include an abnormality in the interleukin-1 receptor antagonist gene, in the tumor necrosis factor alpha gene, and in the endothelial nitric oxide cynthase gene. Studies are under way to determine whether interleukin and/or tumor necrosis factor alpha, in various forms, mitigate the inflammatory response in IBD.

Studies of twins, raised either together or apart, have shown a higher rate of both suffering from IBD when they are monozygotic (having begun life as a single egg) than when they are dizygotic (having begun life as two simultaneously fertilized eggs). This information, along with instances of family members developing the diseases over time in different locations, points to a genetic component.

In addition, IBD is among the diseases often found in people diagnosed with one of three rare genetic syndromes: Turner's syndrome, which also has an autoimmune component; Hermansky-Pudlak syndrome (an autosomal recessive syndrome); and glycogen-storage disease type Ib, which includes an abnormal neutrophil function. Inflammatory bowel disease also has a high rate of association with other immune disorders, many of them with the same kind of familial traits as IBD. Among these are:

Ankylosing spondylitis (AS): approximately 10 percent of those with AS also have IBD, and as many as 10 percent of those with IBD have AS.

Psoriasis: about 10 percent of those with Crohn disease also have psoriasis, and psoriasis is commonly found in the families of those with Crohn disease.

Primary sclerosing cholangitis (PSC): approximately 50–70 percent of those with PSC also have ulcerative colitis.

Multiple sclerosis (MS): a familial concurrence of MS and IBD has been shown, as well as an increased rate of MS in individuals with IBD.

There is also an increased frequency of organ-specific autoimmune disorders (insulin-dependent diabetes, autoimmune thyroid disease, and systemic lupus erythematosus) in individuals with ulcerative colitis.

Because potential inflammatory bowel disease genes have been found on a number of chromosomes, it is speculated that there may be several different genes that predispose an individual to have either ulcerative colitis or Crohn disease.

This fits well with the observation that IBD has different variants, with a number of different clinical and laboratory findings.

Ulcerative proctitis, left-sided ulcerative colitis, ulcerative pancolitis, Crohn colitis, and Crohn disease of the small bowel may, in fact, be distinct diseases. However, there is no evidence of familial pattern in a particular manifestation (i.e., with two first cousins, one might have pan-ulcerative colitis and the other Crohn disease of the ileum and colon).

Infections

Are Crohn disease and ulcerative colitis infectious diseases? Are they the manifestations of systemic responses to acute infectious episodes? Are they the human manifestation of *Mycobacterium paratuberculosis (M. paratuberculosis)*, which causes Johne's (pronounced "yonez") disease in cattle?

Part of the reason it is often difficult to diagnose inflammatory bowel disease is that its symptoms so closely resemble those of a number of other diseases. Crohn disease is so much like ileocecal tuberculosis as to be almost indistinguishable from it. Indeed, before Dr. Burrill Crohn and his colleagues described the entire group of symptoms and found them all in a population, what is now known as Crohn disease was given the diagnosis of tuberculosis. Of course, today, a simple skin test will show whether there are antibodies to the human tuberculosis organism.

M. paratuberculosis infects many mammals, including primates. Both Johne's disease and Crohn disease are epidemic in Scotland. The only thing that keeps Johne's disease from being passed from cows to humans via milk is the pasteurization process. Current theories about the heterogeneity of Crohn disease—there may be many distinct microbacterial or other causes, which combine with one or more susceptible genes—

have led scientists to begin researching *M. paraturberculosis* as a possible triggering event that leads to Crohn disease.

Other potential infectious triggers being studied include *Yersinia enterocolitica,* a bacterial infection, *Chlamydia trachomatis* of the anorectal region, a sexually transmitted bacterial infection, which both resemble Crohn disease, and *Campylobacter* and *Shigella,* two infections often caused by improper or unsanitary food preparation, which both resemble ulcerative colitis.

However, all of the research in this area is retrospective, involving a search for statistical correlations in old data about illness. Even if the number of people who develop clinical symptoms of inflammatory bowel disease after an enteric infection is high, it is not possible to attribute absolute cause and effect. Researchers continue to search for infectious agents that may contribute to either development or progression of Crohn disease or ulcerative colitis.

German researchers recently isolated a microinvasive *E. coli* from colonic biopsies of patients with ulcerative colitis. And in California, researchers have identified genetic material that appears to belong to infectious organisms in the intestinal walls of patients with inflammatory bowel disease. This genetic material was found below the surface-lining cells, the lamina propria. We have always known that bacteria live in the gut, but not that some bore through the intestinal lining into the underlying tissue.

Discovery, however, does not indicate causality. University of North Carolina researchers were able to isolate from the stool of patients with ulcerative colitis two bacterias, *Bacteriodes volgatus* and *E. coli*. They then colonized the bacteria into a germ-free rat. The bacteria did not induce colitis.

Such "blind alleys" are frequent in all medical research. And while the search continues for infectious agents that either cause or contribute to inflammatory bowel disease, to date there is no proven bacterial or viral cause.

Immune Imbalance

Another avenue of research is the attempt to more fully understand the cascade of inflammatory events that occur in response to normal gut bacteria in people with IBD. Those who study the immune issues present in inflammatory bowel disease focus primarily on the immune system of the mucosal lining of the gut. The mucosal immune system is somewhat different from the systemic lymphatic system.

The goal of all of the immunology research is to create better therapies to control the inappropriate immune response, whatever it may be and whatever may be causing it, with fewer side effects than those brought on by currently available medications. Again, a "cure" is not expected from this research in and of itself.

Lymphoid cells make up about 25 percent of all intestinal cells, and the intestine is considered to be a lymphoid organ. It is estimated that the number of microbial cells within the gut at any one time is greater than the total number of cells in the body—one billion to one trillion bacteria per gram of intestinal content. This puts the intestinal immune system in a constant state of work. Some argue that the normal intestine is in a constant state of mild physiologic inflammation.

The immune theory encompasses a number of hypotheses as to how the immune system is responding inappropriately. These are immunodeficiency, autoimmunity and anticolon antibodies, autoimmunity and cells cytotoxic for colonic epithelial cells, and abnormal immunoregulation.

Immunodeficiency

According to one theory of the primary cause of inflammatory bowel disease, a deficiency exists in some aspect of the immune system. Deficiency in cell-mediated immunity, in neutrophils, in macrophages, and in the IgA system have all been postulated. In support of this theory is the fact that those with certain immune deficiencies can have histologic conditions that resemble inflammatory bowel disease.

However, there are many problems with this theory. Only a minority of individuals with Crohn disease or ulcerative colitis show these immune deficiencies. In addition, individuals with inflammatory bowel disease do not have any increased susceptibility to infections by any known viral, bacterial, fungal, or parasitic pathogens. Finally, a number of medications used in successful treatment of inflammatory bowel disease symptoms work by immunosuppression, which is inconsistent with inherent immunodeficiency.

Autoimmunity and Anticolon Antibodies

The notion that inflammatory bowel disease is an autoimmune response is an old one. In ulcerative colitis, which is confined to the epithelium of the colon, antibodies have been found to three colon antigens—serum anticolon lipopolysaccharide; colitis colon-bound antigen (CCA-IgA), and antiepithelial cell-associated components (Anti-ECAC). Two of these three antibodies are also present in Crohn disease; CCA-IgA is not.

Autoimmunity and Cells Cytotoxic for Colonic Epithelial Cells

An autoimmune reaction to the cells of the epithelium within the colon might be involved in the pathogenesis of both ulcerative colitis and Crohn disease. Cytotoxic cells kill other cells, in this case the cells of the epithelial lining of the large intestine.

Cells that are cytotoxic for colonic epithelial cells have been found within the peripheral blood of most individuals with either ulcerative colitis or Crohn disease. These cytotoxic cells are not present in the blood of normal controls, nor are they found in the blood of individuals with a host of other diseases. Such cytotoxic cells are present in the blood during periods of active disease and during remission; however, they are no longer present ten days after resection of damaged tissue.

This theory would be very powerful if cells cytotoxic for colonic epithelial cells were found only in individuals with ulcerative colitis and with Crohn colitis; the presence of such cells in those with Crohn disease of the small intestine makes this theory more problematic. Also, the lack of techniques for maintaining epithelial cells in culture for long periods of time makes this phenomenon difficult to study in the laboratory.

Abnormal Immunoregulation

Another line of inquiry involves the immune system of those affected by Crohn disease or ulcerative colitis and their bodies' inability to regulate immune reaction to normal bacteria that reside in the intestinal lumen. The lumen of the small bowel and colon both contain a large number of various anaerobic bacteria capable of activating mucosal immune cells. Experimental models of IBD introduced into germ-free animals create no chronic gastrointestinal or joint inflammation.

The intestinal system is usually "tolerant" of these normal bacteria, while responding to unknown invaders. In a condition of abnormal immunoregulation, the intestinal immune system loses tolerance for normal bacteria, is activated, and doesn't turn off. Researchers believe there is a genetic predisposition to such an "overeager" immune regulation response.

New Immunoregulatory Medications

Two medications that have shown promise in preventing rejection of transplanted organs are under study for use in battling IBD. Tacrolimus has been tested and appears to be useful in treating acute attacks of IBD that do not respond to steroids. In one small study, eleven patients achieved rapid remission. Mycophenolate mofetil, combined with steroids, has been shown to be effective in small groups of patients with chronic active Crohn disease that has not responded to standard therapy.

In addition to new ones, more established immunoregulatory medications are being used in a novel fashion. Specifically, both 6MP and Imuran have been used successfully to maintain remission in inflammatory bowel disease after a remission induced with cyclosporin.

Leaky Gut

Increased intestinal permeability, sometimes called the "leaky gut syndrome," is a condition in which microscopic breaches occur in the wall of the small intestine. One of the intestine's functions is to allow nutrients to pass into the bloodstream. However, when the intestinal barrier is compromised and the tight junctions of the intestinal epithelium become "leaky," larger molecules can also pass through.

Since 1980, this phenomenon has been studied through the use of permeability probes taken orally. Normally, these probes pass across the intestinal epithelium in very small amounts, if at all. However, in the individual with inflammatory bowel disease, passage increases dramatically.

The important question is whether increased permeability is a cause of inflammatory bowel disease or a symptom of chronic inflammation. In an attempt to answer this, researchers look to compare permeability in individuals encountering a flare-up of inflammatory bowel disease with that of individuals who have inactive inflammatory bowel disease and relatives of individuals with inflammatory bowel disease who do not themselves suffer from either of the diseases.

Those in remission show permeability more closely related to normal controls than to those with active disease. About 90 percent of relatives of individuals with inflammatory bowel disease have permeability similar to normal controls, while about 10 percent have permeability similar to those with diagnosed disease. To learn whether permeability is a precursor to disease, cohorts of relatives who test each way would need to be studied over time to see if those with high permeability had a higher lifetime incidence of inflammatory bowel disease.

Other studies have looked into whether an increase in permeability in individuals who are in medically induced or surgical remission from IBD can be an early warning sign of a flare-up. Intestinal permeability to five grams lactulose and two grams mannitol has been shown to be predictive of flare-up in the first twelve months after the beginning of a remission. Permeability to one hundred grams of sucrose is not predictive, nor is the plasma postheparin diamine oxidase activity. However, even if permeability is a precursor to clinical symptoms of IBD, there is no evidence that it is a cause.

Biological Therapies

In late 1998, the Food and Drug Administration approved the first medication solely for treatment of Crohn disease. The drug, infliximab (trade name Remicade), ushered in a new wave of potential biologic therapies to treat IBD. Infliximab is a chimeric monoclonal antibody, a human-made protein designed to target a specific biological substance—in this case, human tumor necrosis factor alpha (TNF-alpha). TNF, which occurs naturally in the body, has been shown to be one of the major culprits in the intestinal inflammatory process characteristic of IBD.

Remicade was engineered through the use of both mouse and human cells; variable regions of a mouse antihuman TNF monoclonal antibody were combined with human IgG1. Infliximab acts both as a carrier of cytokines (chemicals) and as a TNF antagonist. The net effect is that infliximab renders TNF-alpha biologically inactive.

The FDA approved infliximab for two specific uses. The first is to treat Crohn disease that is refractory to standard treatment and that renders individuals steroid dependent, meaning that a flare-up occurs on successive attempts to taper off steroids. For this purpose, a single two-hour infusion of infliximab is given.

In clinical trials for this use, 48 percent of patients treated with Remicade showed a remission after four weeks, while only 4 percent given a placebo (sugar pill) experienced remission.

Individuals who took part in the clinical trials had to be prednisone dependent, meaning that they were unable to go below twenty milligrams of prednisone daily without recurrence of severe symptoms. The individuals stayed on their steroid dose for the duration of the treatment with Remicade. Because of this, it is not known whether infliximab is truly "steroid sparing." Further studies will look at whether infliximab is effective without concurrent steroid use.

The second use is to help close draining enterocutaneous fistulas—fistulas between the intestine and the skin of the abdomen or between the rectum and the perianal area that drain pus and bowel contents. Enterocutaneous fistulas are painful infections that often do not respond to high-dose antibiotics. For this treatment, a three-infusion regimen is undertaken, with the second infusion two weeks after the first and the third four weeks after the second.

Studies completed in 1999 show good results. Most, and in some cases all, draining fistulas were closed following three injections of five milligrams per kilo of body weight; there was less success when ten milligrams per kilo were used. Only 6 percent of study participants experienced side effects, including headache, low-grade fever, dizziness, and flushing, usually during or immediately after injection.

A large study begun in 1999 is looking at the effectiveness in maintaining closure of enterocutaneous fistulas when reinfusion is done every two months. No data exists yet on the potential side effects, as well as the effectiveness, of long-term use of infliximab.

Two other anti-TNF substances, CDP571, a humanized monoclonal antibody, and Etanercept, a human fusion protein, are also under study.

One small trial of CDP571 had been reported by mid 1999. In it, twenty individuals with moderate Crohn disease were given five milligrams per kilogram of body weight of CDP571, and ten were given placebo. At two weeks after receiving CDP571, the mean reduction in the Crohn Disease Activity Index (CDAI) was nearly 100 points, from 263 to 167. The placebo group had no significant change in its mean index score, from 253 to 247. (A person with a CDAI score of under 150 is considered to be in remission, and one who is above 450 is considered critically ill.)

Infliximab and CDP571 have been studied in ulcerative colitis as well. Neither has been approved by the FDA.

No studies have been reported on Etanercept for use in either Crohn disease or ulcerative colitis. However, Etanercept has produced results in the treatment of rheumatoid arthritis, which has been shown to be closely linked with IBD by similarities in the cascade of immune response, by the number of people who suffer from both conditions, and by the number of families in which individuals have one or the other condition.

In studies of Etanercept for rheumatoid arthritis, 71 percent of those who took twenty-five milligrams of Etanercept twice weekly showed clinical improvement, against 25 percent on placebo. Infliximab and CDP571 have also been studied in rheumatoid arthritis. None of these has yet been approved by the FDA for this use.

Another biologic approach to influence the production of inflammatory cytokines has recently been used. The agent thalidomide has been shown to decrease production of both tumor necrosis factor alpha and interleukin-12. Small studies from both Cedars-Sinai Hospital in California and the University of Chicago have suggested that thalidomide may be effective in treatment of Crohn disease.

Any use of thalidomide would be controversial. Prescribed in Canada and Europe in the late 1950s and early 1960s as an antinausea medicine for morning sickness in pregnant women, thalidomide was taken off the market after being shown to cause severe birth defects. The drug was never approved in the United States; consequently, few "thalidomide babies" were born in this country. Children born to mothers who had used thalidomide often had stunted arms and legs, severe complications of the hip and shoulder joints, and few fingers or toes, if they had distinguishable hands or feet. Today, thalidomide is approved for very limited use in individuals with Hanson's disease, otherwise known as leprosy. It is the most tightly controlled drug on the market; a woman of childbearing age who accepts a prescription for thalidomide must agree to use contraceptives, to have a monthly pregnancy test, and to undergo a therapeutic abortion should she become pregnant while using the medication.

Another novel biologic agent is alpha-4 integrin, which promotes the migration of inflammatory cells across blood vessel lining. A group of doctors in the United Kingdom treated patients with Crohn disease with an antibody against alpha-4 integrin, and demonstrated a possible biologic affect. The dose studied was too small to induce remission; experiments with higher doses will take place if safety data from this study warrant.

Other biologic treatments under study include antibodies to block cytokines that promote inflammation. Studies of interleukin-10 and interleukin-12 for people with active Crohn disease have been conducted since 1997, and a study of antibodies targeted against interleukin-12 for refractory Crohn disease began in 1999.

Antisense oglionucleotides are also under study for treatment of refractory Crohn disease. An agent that aims to block the genetic messages that instruct intercellular adhesion molecule-1 (ICAM-1), a molecule that increases and prolongs the inflammatory response in people with IBD, has been studied in a small group of twenty steroid-dependent people with Crohn disease.

Removal of Inflammatory Cells

Another approach to influencing the inflammatory reaction (rather than using agents to turn off inflammation) is to experiment with a technique to remove inflammatory cells from the body. These techniques, which are variously called extracorporeal photochemotherapy, phyta therapy, and leukophoresis, have been tried in several research centers with some success in the treatment of inflammatory bowel disease.

Other Research into New Medications

The following are among other medications being studied.

Omega-3 fatty acids, such as those found in fish oils, may reduce the level of leukotrienes, which play a role in inflammation. Small studies show some improvement in people with active ulcerative colitis, although not in maintaining remission in colitis. Another study showed that omega-3 fatty acids did maintain remission in those with Crohn disease.

Short-chain fatty acids (SCFAs), such as butyrate, exist in the lining of the colon. These nutrients are produced during digestion of complex carbohydrates. The intestinal lining of individuals with ulcerative colitis may not produce these nutrients. In several small trials, thirty-five of a total of forty-one individuals benefited from SCFA enemas. SCFAs may also be useful for treatment of pouchitis (inflammation of the internal pouch surgically created to collect stool in those who have had their colon removed and the ileum reconnected to the rectum so they can defecate naturally).

Bowman-Birk protease inhibitor, which has been shown to prevent cancer in animals, is being studied for use in ulcerative colitis. The risk of colon cancer increases over time in those who have ulcerative colitis.

Heparin, a blood thinner, has shown some effectiveness in refractory ulcerative colitis. Heparin may interfere with cytokines that cause inflammation. Heparin may also affect the vascular endothelium itself. A recent trial suggested that heparin, in addition to being safe for use in patients with ulcerative colitis, may even provide some benefit to them.

Rapidly metabolized corticosteroids such as budesonide are being looked at as a way of maintaining steroid therapy for those who become steroid dependent, while reducing the side effects and long-term risks of more traditional steroids. These drugs are quickly cleared from the bloodstream, and have shown results similar to prednisone in inducing remission in both Crohn disease and ulcerative colitis. Budesonide is currently available in some countries—although not in the United States—both as a capsule and as an enema preparation. Work is also being done on a delayed-release capsule to treat ileal disease in patients with Crohn disease.

Probiotic agents (beneficial bacteria) are being examined both as a way to replace toxic bacteria after antibiotic treatment and a way to release protective chemicals. Substances such as lactobacilli have shown results in animal studies, as well as in one small study of individuals with recurrent pouchitis.

Nicotine is also being studied. Although most individuals with ulcerative colitis are nonsmokers, a higher proportion of newly diagnosed patients are former smokers who had quit within the four years before diagnosis. Nicotine has been shown to be protective in ulcerative colitis (although harmful in Crohn disease). It has been demonstrated that nicotine, used in chewing gum and patch form, is effective in treatment of active colitis, although not in maintaining remission. A number of individuals in all studies have suffered nicotine side effects, mostly headaches, lightheadedness, nausea, and sleep disturbance. Nicotine enemas have also been attempted for those with mild-to-moderate proctosigmoiditis. Both self-reported and sigmoidascopic symptoms were reduced in many patients, without any nicotine side effects.

Appendix A: Organizations

The best resource for information about Crohn disease and ulcerative colitis is the Crohn's & Colitis Foundation of America (CCFA). CCFA's national headquarters is:

386 Park Avenue South
17th Floor
New York, NY 10016–8804
(212) 685–3440
(800) 932–2423
www.ccfa.org

CCFA has chapters in most states and more than one chapter in some states. The national headquarters can give you the phone number and contact name for the chapter nearest you. Chapters hold informational and educational meetings and facilitate support groups for people who live with inflammatory bowel disease, as well as for spouses, parents of children with IBD, and other interested groups. Chapters also sponsor social events, as well as fundraising activities to support the local chapter and the national research and education efforts.

CCFA's Web page was given awards for both design and content in 1997 and 1998. You can register to join the organization via the Web, ask questions of experts using the organization's Web-linked e-mail system, and read the most up-to-date news and research reports about IBD.

For those who have had surgery that includes an ostomy, the United Ostomy Association should also be helpful:

United Ostomy Association
19772 McArthur Blvd., Suite 200
Irvine, CA 92612–2405
(800) 826–0826
www.uao.org

Appendix B: Books

About Crohn Disease and Ulcerative Colitis in General

The Angry Gut, W. Grant Thompson (Plenum Press, 1993).
Crohn's Disease & Ulcerative Colitis, Fred Saibil (Firefly Books, 1997).
Inflammatory Bowel Disease: A Guide for Patients and Their Families, Staney H. Stein and Richard P. Rood, editors (Lippincott-Raven, 1999).

About Nutrition for Those with Inflammatory Bowel Disease

Breaking the Vicious Cycle: Intestinal Health through Diet, Elaine Gottschall (Kirkton Press Ltd. [Canada], 1995).
Eating Right for a Bad Gut: The Complete Nutritional Guide to Ileitis, Colitis, Crohn's Disease and Inflammatory Bowel Disease, James Scala (Plume, 1992).
The IBD Nutrition Book, Jan K. Greenwood (John Wiley & Sons, 1992).

About Chronic Illness

Meeting the Challenge: Living with Chronic Illness, Audrey Kron (self-published, 1996 [call 248–626-6960 to order]).
Young People and Chronic Illness (True Stories, Help, and Hope), Kelly Huegel (Free Spirit Publishing, 1998).

About the Difficulties of Steroid Treatment

Coping with Prednisone (and Other Cortisone-Related Medicines), Eugenia Zuckerman and Julie R. Ingelfinger (St. Martin, 1997).

Personal Stories

Alive & Kicking, Rolf Benirschke and Mike Yorkey (Firefly Books, 1996).

Colitis (The Experience of Illness), Michael P. Kelly (Tavistock, 1992).

Patient Power: Overcoming Chronic Illness, James Marshall Galbraith (Benchmark Books, 1998).

Second Act : Life After Colostomy, Barbara Barrie (Scribner, 1997).

Appendix C: Other Web Sites

Because the Web is constantly changing, the best way to get to the newest, most exciting Web pages is to do a search. Simply ask your browser to search "Crohn's" or "colitis." In January 1999, a search of the word "Crohn's" found that the top 10 matches had 3,534 hits. A large number of these were personal Web pages created by newly diagnosed individuals wanting to set up communication links to others, then creating resource guides from all of the responses they got (many were not very good).

Another way to do it is to go to the IBD Home Page, www.kitsap.net/health/ccl, which in January 1999 listed about 25 other sites that you can get into simply by clicking the link. Among these sites were those of the Cleveland Clinic Department of Colo-Rectal surgery and the UCLA Digestive Diseases Center. Others included such specialized sites as the J-Pouch Home Page and the enjoyable IBD Humor Page.

One site definitely worth a look is Keith's Crohn's Chronical, a graphics-heavy on-line newspaper devoted to the support of Crohn's patients. This site is best viewed with Netscape.

Note to the Reader

We are interested in learning from you about your experiences with inflammatory bowel disease. If you are interested and willing, we would share your experiences and those of your family in subsequent editions of this book.

What have you learned over the years that has been particularly helpful to you? What advice or services have you found particularly useful to you and your family? What do you wish had been better explained to you earlier in the course of your living with IBD?

Also, if we can answer any questions, feel free to contact us. We can be reached at:

Ronald J. Vender M.D.
Gastroenterology Center of Connecticut
2200 Whitney Avenue Suite 360
Hamden CT 06518

Jon Zonderman
535 Howellton Road
Orange CT 06477

Glossary

Abscess A localized collection of inflammatory cells (pus) that can occur in acute or chronic infections. In those with IBD, it tends to occur outside the bowel wall or around the anal canal. An abscess can be drained surgically, although sometimes it responds to antibiotic treatment.

Adhesions Thin fibrous bands of scar tissue in the abdominal cavity that typically result from an earlier infection or surgery. When the adhesions connect loops of bowel together or cause partial blockage of the bowel, pain and vomiting can occur. Adhesions may require surgical correction.

Anastomosis The connection of two vessels. In IBD, the surgical joining of the ends of healthy bowel after a diseased segment has been removed.

Autoimmunity A condition in which the body's immune system reacts to its own tissues.

Colectomy The removal of all or part of the large bowel (total colectomy or subtotal colectomy).

Colostomy A surgical opening connecting the colon to the surface of the body allowing for elimination of waste.

Complementary (alternative) medicine The addition to standard medical care of medical techniques that fall outside the Western scientific tradition.

Endoscopy The examination of the inside of one of the hollow organs of the gastrointestinal tract with a special instrument known as an endoscope. A flexible tube with a camera lens is either passed through the patient's mouth for an examination of the upper GI system or inserted into the anal canal for an examination of the lower GI system. Endoscopic examination of the first sixty centimeters of the colon can be accomplished with a sigmoidoscope, or examination of the entire colon can be accomplished with a colonoscope.

Epidemiology The study of frequency, distribution, and causes of disease in populations.

Exacerbation An increase in the severity of a disease, manifested by an increase either in symptoms or in signs.

Extraintestinal manifestations Signs or symptoms of disease that appear outside the gastrointestinal tract; IBD examples include joint pain and inflammation, eye pain and inflammation, and skin lesions.

Fissure A deep cleft or slit. The term is commonly used to describe a slit in the tissue lining the anal canal, which can be extremely painful and difficult to treat.

Fistula An abnormal connection between two surfaces. In IBD, this can lead to an inappropriate opening between two different loops of bowel, or between the bowel and another internal organ such as the bladder, or between the bowel and the outside of the abdominal wall.

Idiopathic Of unknown cause.

Ileostomy A surgical opening connecting the ileum to the surface of the abdomen and allowing for the elimination of waste.

Immunology Study of the response of the body to invasion by material that is not "self."

Inflammation The body's response to an injury or irritation caused by infection or by physical or chemical agents. The body's immune system responds, leading to redness, heat, pain, and swelling.

Laboratory evidence Results of laboratory tests.

Lactose intolerance The inability to digest the milk sugar lactose, resulting from an absence or low production of the enzyme lactase. This disorder is characterized by cramps and diarrhea after the consumption of food that contains lactose, such as milk or ice cream.

Lumen The space in the interior of the intestine and other hollow organs.

Obstruction A partial or complete blockage of the intestine. This can be the result of inflammation and swelling, scar tissue, or food trapped in a narrowed segment. The obstruction can be caused by internal narrowing or an external blockage, such as an adhesion.

Oxalate stones A form of kidney stones formed by the chemical calcium oxalate. Oxalate is found in many plants.

Perforation An abnormal opening in the bowel wall that allows bowel contents to leak into the abdominal cavity.

Peristalsis A wave-like smooth-muscle movement that allows food to be transported downward through the gastrointestinal tract.

Radiologic signs Areas of diseased tissue that can be seen with the use of radiological exam techniques such as barium enema or small-bowel series.

Remission The time when an individual is free of disease. In a clinical remission, the person will have no clinical symptoms, although laboratory evidence and radiological signs of disease may still be present. In a complete remission, all evidence of disease is inactive, including both symptoms and signs.

Resection The surgical removal of a section or all of a structure.

Sign Objective evidence of disease as perceived by a physician or other examiner.

Stricture A localized narrowing of a hollow organ such as the bowel. The stricture can be caused by inflammation with swelling or by scar tissue built up from repeated active disease and healing. Strictures can be surgically resected or opened.

Symptoms A sensation or change in function experienced by a patient.

Index